Low dose medicine

Healing without side effects using low dose homeopathic cytokines, hormones, and neurotrophines

Low dose medicine

Healing without side effects using low dose homeopathic cytokines, hormones, and neurotrophines

Max Corradi

Jaborandi Publishing

Other books by the author:

Healing with Micotherapy
Self-Healing with Therapeutic Mushrooms
Jaborandi Publishing

Cures without side effects
Practical healing manual of the most essential and effective
biotherapy treatments
Jaborandi Publishing

CONTENTS

Chapter 4   56

Low dose growth factors and their main indications   56

Chapter 5   61

Chapter 7

Low dose medicine general treatment protocols

This book is dedicated to all the great healers that work for the benefit of beings.

Important Disclaimer:

The informational knowledge presented in this book is intended to complement medical treatment and not to replace conventional medicine or the advice of your doctor.
Always seek professional help.

NOTHING CONTAINED IN THIS BOOK IS INTENDED TO BE NOR CAN IT BE TAKEN FOR MEDICAL DIAGNOSIS OR TREATMENT

Introduction

In my book 'Cures without side effects' I have introduced the concept of healing without side effects using the power of the subconscious mind and natural medicine.

In part one of that book I have described the Biotherapy system and the homeopathic and herbal remedies which can be employed in order to heal oneself without any side effects.

Moreover, in that book I have also introduced and explained, somewhat succinctly, the concept of using low dose homeopathic cytokines, hormones and growth factors in order to re-program and regulate deranged biochemical pathways.

This book covers in much more detail how to use this new form of therapy called 'low dose medicine' or 'physiological regulating medicine', and in particular, how to heal oneself using low dose homeopathic cytokines, interleukins, neurotransmitters, neurotrophines, hormones and growth factors.

The aim of this book is to be at the same time a manual and also a compendium to my book 'Cures without side effects' describing possible different ways to cure oneself without side effects.

Part 1

Low dose medicine, cytokines, hormones, and neurotrophines

Chapter 1

What is low dose medicine?

Low dose medicine is a new therapeutic approach which aims at restoring physiology through communicating or signaling molecules such as cytokines, interleukins, growth factors, neuropeptides, neurotransmitters and hormones prepared in low dose-active dilutions (through the homeopathic method of dilution and succussion) and therefore without side effects. (For more information about classic homeopathy and the 'homeopathic processing' of dilution and dynamization see my book 'Cures without side effects').

Since these molecules have the same physiological concentration (nanograms to picograms) as the molecules present in our organism which control and regulate organic functions under healthy conditions, one could define low dose medicine as 'physiological regulating medicine' but also as 'preventive medicine' since low dose active preparations have virtually no side effects.

Low dose medicine is also in many cases a resolutive therapy because it works on the whole organism directly by using molecules which work at the cellular level in order to re-direct biochemical pathways when these are deranged or inhibited.

By using low dose medicine one can act directly on the PNEI (Psycho-Neuro-Endocrine-Immunitary) system with the aim of regulating cell's activity, when this is inhibited or disturbed by endogenous or exogenous stressors. At this level one is able to restore the capacities for cellular self-regulation which are indispensable for maintaining homeostasis *(for more information on the PNEI system see related section in this book and my book 'Cures without side effects').*

Recent findings have shown that cytokines, interleukins, hormones, growth factors and neuropeptides correctly diluted and dynamized become active, through a mechanism of sensitization and activation of cellular receptors.

As we will see in the therapeutic strategy, one of the best way to correct a deficiency is to provide low (activated) doses of the same substance to stimulate its metabolism and physiologic production, and the result of the action of these low dose active molecules is a physiological modulation and regulation of the biochemical pathways when these are deranged or inhibited.

In a nutshell, low dose medicine can be defined as an up-to-date integration of homeopathy, Psycho-Neuro-Endocrine-Immunology (PNEI) and molecular biology.

The therapeutic strategy

In general low dose medicine should be used according to the following decisional process:

- If the pathological condition is the expression of a down-regulation (deficiency) of a certain molecule (cytokine, interleukin, hormone, neuropeptide, neurotransmitter, growth factor), the same low dose molecule will be **used in order to stimulate (up-regulate) its physiological production.**
- If the pathological condition is the expression of an up-regulation (excess) of a certain molecule (cytokine, interleukin, hormone, neuropeptide, neurotransmitter) **the 'opposing low dose molecule' will be used in order to down- regulate its physiological production.**
- According to a more 'symptoms oriented decisional processes' where the low dose molecules are **prescribed to suit and to manage the particular symptoms of the disease.**
- In combination with classic homeopathic single and/or complex remedies in order to achieve a faster remission

- In addition to conventional standard medications with the aim of counteracting their side effects or in order to reduce the dosage and frequency of the medication.

General dosage: the daily dose is 15 to 20 drops in little mineral water to be taken twice a day, and kept under the tongue for deep absorption before swallowing, for periods ranging from 3 to 6 weeks or longer, and according to the particular condition and individual reaction.

Chapter 2

What are cytokines?

Cytokines can be described as small messenger and signaling molecules released by cells that have a specific effect on the interactions between cells, on the communication between cells and on the behavior of cells.

The term 'cytokine' encompasses a large and diverse family of messenger and signaling molecules produced throughout the body by cells of diverse embryological origin. There is no general agreement as to which molecules should be termed cytokine, and part of this difficulty in distinguishing cytokines from other molecules, is that some of the immunomodulating effects of cytokines are systemic, meaning that they act on the whole body system rather than on a localized system or organ.

Cytokines were officially recognized in 1979 and this discovery created a revolution in immunology and medicine in general. Since then, an enormous amount of research has been devoted to cytokines.

Cytokines are critical to the development and functioning of both the innate and adaptive immune response, they are often secreted by immune cells that have encountered a pathogen, thereby activating and recruiting further immune cells to increase the system's response to the pathogen.

Although pivotal in triggering and regulating the immune response, they are not limited to the immune system alone, in fact many cytokines are now known to be produced by cells other than immune cells and they can have effects on non-immune cells as well.

Cytokines are also involved in several developmental processes during embryo genesis. **The complex network of cytokines balances pro-inflammatory and anti-inflammatory** effects, and an imbalance between pro- and anti-inflammatory cytokines or the uncontrolled production of cytokines can result in chronic inflammatory disease, allergies or auto-immune disease.

Broadly speaking, cytokines can include different types of molecules like 'monokines' produced by mononuclear phagocytic cells, 'chemokines' produced by many kinds of leukocytes and other cell types, 'lymphokines' produced by activated lymphocytes (especially T helper cells), 'interleukins' that act as mediators between leukocytes, 'peptides' (cell signaling molecules), 'growth factors' which promote cell growth and 'interferons' (INF) which respond to infected cells and cancer cells.

We could also divide cytokines according to their biological role such as growth factors which promote cell growth proliferation and differentiation, interleukins and lymphokines which are capable of creating a communicating network within the immune system, and chemokines and lymphokines which are mainly involved in inflammation.

Unfortunately cytokines used by immunologists and other medical specialists in conventional medicine are in pharmacological doses and have very strong and sometimes lethal side-effects.

In low dose medicine, on the other hand, cytokines are used in low 'activated' doses without any side effects and with the therapeutic concept of modulating and regulating cell activity and cell communication and restoring natural physiology.

Low dose cytokines have the same physiological concentration (nanograms to picograms) as the molecules present in our organism and work through a mechanism of sensitization and activation of cellular receptors.

The result of the action of these low dose cytokines is a physiological modulation of the system cell's activity and restoration of the capacity for cellular self-regulation.

Cytokine storm

A common mistake people usually make is to try to 'boost' one's immune system through the use of herbal or nutraceutical remedies with the idea of fighting off an infection, but in fact **an over reacting immune system can sometimes be the cause of an over-secretion of cytokines which can trigger a dangerous syndrome known as a 'cytokine storm'.**

Cytokine storms have the potential to do significant damage to body tissues and organs. If a cytokine storm occurs in the lungs, for example, fluids and immune cells such as macrophages may accumulate and eventually block off the airways, potentially resulting in death.

Cytokine storms were the main cause of death in the 1918 'Spanish Flu' pandemic, the 2003 SARS (caused by coronavirus) and the Avian Flu (A/H5N1) virus in 2008. Deaths were weighted more heavily towards people with healthy immune systems, due to its ability to produce stronger immune responses, with increasing cytokine levels.

By using low dose cytokines, on the other hand, one can up-regulate or down-regulate, if needed, the immune system responses without any side-effects according to each individual case, resulting in a perfect modulation of all immune processes during an infection outbreak.

Recombinant cytokines

The cytokines used in low dose medicine are called 'recombinant cytokines' and are the same as the ones used by specialists and immunologists in conventional medicine, with the enormous difference that in low dose medicine these recombinant cytokines are then properly diluted and activated through a process called 'succussion' to avoid any side-effects (*for the homeopathic method of dilution and succession see my book 'Cures without side effects*).

Recombinant cytokines are mostly produced by expression from suitable cloning vectors containing the desired cytokine gene, including 'Escherichia coli', 'Pichia pastoris', 'Baculovirus' and 'Poxvirus' systems which can be expressed in yeast, mammalian (human) cells or insect cell systems.

Expression in each system results in a protein that differs, to a varying extent, from the native molecules. The expression system can influence the pharmacokinetic properties, biologic activity, and clinical toxicity of recombinant proteins.

The 'Pichia pastoris' expression system seem to be particularly well suited for the production of recombinant cytokines because the yeast cells are not a source of endogenous toxins, as for example is the case with E. coli.

Recombinant human cytokines (produced from human cells) are more authentic in terms of both physical properties and biochemical functions, however, the current process of human cell expression requires a large quantity of DNA and medium supplemented with bovine serum with increasing costs.

Another emerging technology for the production of recombinant cytokines is the 'plant-based processing'. Recent development of DNA recombination and plant transformation techniques resulted in creating the novel protein production platforms based on either whole plants or plant cells. The process of using plant-based systems as highly effective production platforms is named 'molecular farming', while the pharmaceutical products obtained in the plant-based systems are often called plant-made pharmaceuticals (PMPs).

Whatever the source of the recombinant cytokine is, in low dose medicine the signaling molecule undergoes a process of dilution and activation and is therefore rendered highly active and, at the same time, harmless in terms of side-effects, not to mention the incredible reduction of costs for the end user.

Pro and anti-inflammatory cytokines

Cytokines are commonly classified into pro-inflammatory and anti-inflammatory, **although recent studies have proven that this distinction is far too simplistic as there are numerous examples illustrating that a given cytokine may behave as a pro as well as anti-inflammatory** depending on the cytokine amount released, the nature of the target cell, the nature of the activating signal and even on the temporal sequence of several cytokines acting on the same cell.

Recent findings from a wide range of cytokine investigations indicate that the net effect of the inflammatory response is determined by a delicate balance between pro and anti-inflammatory cytokines acting in synergy to coordinate the immune response initiated upon an external signal, and that any perturbation in this equilibrium can drive the host immune response either towards chronic inflammation or towards healing.

Despite what has just been said, we can generally list some of the cytokines which behave as pro or anti-inflammatory. Among the **inflammatory cytokines** according to the severity of the inflammatory response we can list:

Interleukin 1 alpha and beta (IL-1α and IL-1β)
Interleukin 6 (IL- 6)
Tumor necrosis factor α (TNF- α)
Interleukin 8 (IL- 8)
Interleukin 12 (IL- 12)
Interleukin 17 (IL -17)
Interleukin 18 (IL -18)
Interleukin 23 (IL -23)
Granulocyte-macrophage colony stimulating factor (GM-CSF)
Interferon gamma- (IFN- γ)
Ciliary Neurotrophic Factor (CNTF)

Anti-inflammatory or immunoregulatory cytokines that counteract various aspects of the inflammatory response include the following in order of importance of inhibition of pro-inflammatory cytokines:

Anti- interleukin 1 (Anti-IL1)
Interleukin 10 (IL- 10)
Interleukin 4 (IL- 4)
Transforming growth factor-beta (TGF-beta)
Interleukin 11 (IL- 11)
Interleukin 13 (IL- 13)
Interleukin 35 (IL- 35)

Interaction between cytokines and innate and adaptive immunity

In humans two main types of immunity are recognized: the innate (non-specific) and the adaptive (also known as acquired) immunity. Both innate and adaptive immunity depend on the ability of the immune system to distinguish between self and non-self molecules (pathogens).

If a pathogen such as a bacteria or virus manages to breach the layered defenses such as the physical barriers of the skin, the innate immune system provides an immediate, but non-specific response. If the pathogen then successfully evades the innate response, vertebrates possess a second layer of protection called the adaptive immune system which is activated by the innate response.

The innate immune system is the dominant system of defense in most organisms and it is found in all plants and animals.

The innate immune system is non-specific, its response comes into play immediately or within hours of an antigen's appearance in the body in a very effective way but does not confer long lasting immunity against such a pathogen since it lacks an immunological memory.

Cells of the innate immune system include phagocytes cells such as monocytes and macrophages (white blood cells that engulf and absorb waste material, harmful micro organisms or other foreign bodies), and also natural killer (NK) cells, basophils, mast cells, eosinophils and dendritic cells.

Cytokines released from innate immune cells play a key role in the regulation of the immune response.

Cytokines secreted by different innate immune cells includes tumor necrosis factor (TNF), interleukins IL-1, IL-6, IL-10, IL-12, IL-15, and IL-18, interferons such as IFN-α, IFN-β and IFN- γ.

The adaptive (acquired) immune system, on the other hand, allows for a stronger immune response as well as an immunological memory which is maintained by 'memory cells'.

This highly effective specificity allows for the generation of responses that are tailored to specific pathogens or pathogen-infected cells.

Cells that make up the adaptive immune system include the B and T lymphocytes which are derived from hematopoietic stem cells in the bone marrow.

B lymphocytes are involved in the humoral immune response whose primary function is the production of antibodies, whereas T lymphocytes differentiate into different subtypes like the T cytotoxic (Tc) cells, T helper (Th) cells, natural killer T cells (NKT cells).

Cytokines that play a role in the adaptive immune system include interleukins IL-2, IL-4, IL-5, IL-10, IL-12, TGF-β and IFN- γ.

Interaction between cytokines and T lymphocytes

As we have seen, T lymphocytes are a type of white blood cell that plays a central role in adaptive immunity which, once activated, divide rapidly and secrete cytokines which regulate and assist all immune responses.

They are distinguished from other lymphocytes, such as B cells and natural killer cells (NK cells) by the presence of a T-cell receptor (TCR) on their surface and **they are called T cells because they mature in the thymus** (whereas B cells migrate to mature in secondary lymphoid tissues such as the spleen, lymph nodes, Peyer's patches).

Within the T lymphocyte group we can distinguish various subgroups of cells like T helper cells (Th1, Th2, Th3 and Th17), T cytotoxic (Tc) cells, regulatory cells (T reg cells) and Natural Killer T (NKT) cells (not be confused with Natural Killer or NK cells of the innate immune system) which bridge the adaptive immune system with the innate immune system.

Among these different T lymphocyte subgroups, of particular importance are the T helper (Th) lymphocytes also known as CD4+ T cells (because they express the CD4 glycoprotein on their surface) **and also the T cytotoxic (Tc) lymphocytes** also known as CD8+ T cells (since they express the CD8 glycoprotein at their surface).

Moreover, as we will see in the next chapter, T helper (Th) cells are categorized into several subtypes including Th1, Th2, Th3 and Th17.

Interaction between cytokines and T helper (Th) lymphocytes

In general, T helper (Th) cells are important because they assist all other white blood cells immunological processes, including maturation of B cells into plasma cells and memory B cells, and activation of T cytotoxic (Tc) cells and macrophages.

T helper 1 cells (Th1) are the immunity effectors against intracellular pathogens (viruses and bacteria inside host cells) by promoting a cellular immune response.

They are triggered by interleukin IL-2, IL-12, interferon gamma (IFN-γ) and they activate macrophages as well as T cytotoxic cells,

Natural Killer (NK) cells and interferon gamma (IFN-γ) to kill intracellular organisms.

Low dose cytokines which up-regulate Th1 lymphocytes include interleukins IL2, IL12, IFN γ, and the hormone melatonin. There are also some mushrooms such as Ganoderma and Coriolus which stimulate Th1 cell mediated immunity.

Low dose cytokines which down regulate Th1 cells are mainly interleukin IL 4 and IL10 and the hormones cortisol and ACTH.

Th2 cells (Th2) are the immunity effectors against parasitic infection and toxins and promote a humoral immune response.

They are triggered by interleukin 4 (IL-4) and their effector cytokines are IL-4, IL-5, and IL-13. Their main effector cells are eosinophils, basophils, and mast cells and they also help B cells to secrete protective antibodies.

Th2 cells over activation stimulate mast cells to release histamine and are the cause of IgE mediated allergic reactions and hypersensitivity including allergic rhinitis, atopic dermatitis, and asthma.

Low dose cytokines which up-regulate Th2 lymphocytes include interleukins IL4, IL5, IL10, IL13 and the hormones cortisol and ACTH.

Low dose cytokines which down regulate Th2 cells are mainly interleukin IL2, IL12, IFN γ and the hormone melatonin.

Th17 cells (Th17) are a subset of T helper cells which mediate immunity against extracellular bacteria and fungi. They are considered developmentally distinct from Th1 and Th2 cells and an **excessive amount of Th 17 cells are thought to play a key role in autoimmune diseases** such as multiple sclerosis (MS), psoriasis, autoimmune uveitis, diabetes type 1, rheumatoid arthritis (RA), and Crohn's disease.

IL1, IL-6 and IL 23 are thought to drive differentiation into Th17 cells and the effector cytokines associated with Th17 are IL-17, IL1, IL-21, IL-22 and TNF alpha.

Low dose cytokines which up-regulate Th17 lymphocytes include interleukins IL-6, IL 17, IL 21, IL 23 and also TGF-β.

Low dose cytokines which down regulate Th17 cells are mainly interleukin IL4 and IFN γ.

Th3 cells have suppressive/regulatory properties which control auto-aggressive immune responses, they assist mucosal immunity and are involved in protecting mucosal surfaces in the gut from nonpathogenic antigens. They mediate and regulate anti-inflammatory environment by secreting TGF-beta, IL-4 and IL-10. Th3 cells inhibit Th1 and Th2 cells.

Low dose cytokines which up-regulate Th3 are interleukin IL10 and TGF-β.

Interaction between cytokines and T regulatory (Treg) lymphocytes

Regulatory T cells (Treg), formerly known as **suppressor T cells**, are a subpopulation of T cells which modulate the immune system, maintain tolerance to self-antigens, and abrogate autoimmune disease.

Treg cells do not prevent initial T cell activation but rather inhibit a sustained response preventing chronic and potentially damaging pathological responses like self-reactivity, autoimmunity. Treg cells suppress both Th1 and Th2 responses.

Low dose cytokines which up-regulate Treg cells are interleukin IL10 and TGF-β.

The Th1/Th2 driven immune response in relations to common ailments

A healthy immune system is both balanced and dynamic switching back and forth between the Th1 and Th2 driven immune responses as needed, and this allows for a quick eradication of any threat and a return to balance before responding to the next threat.

The inability to respond adequately with a Th1 response and therefore an overactive Th2 response can result in chronic viral infections, AIDS, chronic fatigue syndrome, Candida yeast infections, multiple allergies, asthma, multiple chemical sensitivities (MCS), atopic dermatitis, scleroderma, viral hepatitis and other related illnesses and cancer.

Factors which contribute to induce a Th2 switch and suppress cell-mediated immunity are: vaccinations, heated vegetable oils high in trans-fatty acids, glucose (white sugar), asbestos, lead, mercury and other heavy metals, pesticides, air and water pollutants, morphine, tobacco, the hormone cortisol (due to prolonged stress), HIV, Candida yeast infections, HCV, E-coli, UV-B light, alcohol, sedentary lifestyle, negative mind attitudes, low body temperature, chronic insomnia, weight lifting, and steroids (for muscle gain).

An overactive Th1 response, on the other hand, can worsen already activated (Th17 driven) auto immune diseases like rheumatoid arthritis, multiple sclerosis, diabetes type 1, psoriasis, Chron 's disease, alopecia, vitiligo and most autoimmune endocrine pathologies.

Interaction between cytokines and T cytotoxic (Tc) lymphocytes

Cytotoxic T cells (also known as CD8+ T cells or killer T cell) are cells specialized in killing cancer cells, virus, bacteria and protozoan infected cells or cells that are damaged in other ways.

Low dose cytokines which up-regulate cytotoxic T cells are interleukin IL2, IL12, IFN-α, IFN-γ, and TNF α.

Low dose cytokines which down regulate cytotoxic T cells are mainly interleukin IL10 and TGF-β.

Interaction between cytokines and Natural killer (NK) cells and lymphokine-activated killer (LAK) cells

Natural killer cells (also known as NK cells) are a type of lymphocyte which evolves from lymphoid stem cells and are a major component of the innate immune system.

Their main role is to contain viral infections while the adaptive immune response is generating antigen-specific cytotoxic T cells that can clear the infection, and they also play a major role in the host defense and destruction of both cancer cells and all kinds of mutated cells. They differentiate and mature in the bone marrow, lymph node, spleen, tonsils and thymus from where they enter into the blood stream.

NK cells are activated in response to interferons or macrophage-derived cytokines.

Low dose cytokines which up-regulate NK cells are interleukin IL 2, IL7, IL 12, IL 15, IL 18, IFN-α and IFN γ and the hormone melatonin (there are also mushrooms which stimulate NK cells like Ganoderma lucidum and Coriolus versicolor).

Lymphokine-activated killer cells (or LAK cells) are a type of white blood cell that are produced to kill tumor cells.

Lymphocytes exposed to IL 2, are capable of destroying cancer cells, both primary and metastatic. The mechanism of LAK cells is distinctive from that of natural killer (NK) cells because they can destroy cells that NK cells cannot, moreover, LAK cells are specific to tumor cells and do not display activity against normal cells.

Low dose cytokines which up-regulate LAK cells are interleukin IL 2 and IL7.

Hormones and cytokines cross regulation

Hormones can influence cytokines levels and create a connection between the endocrine system and the immune system.

Female sexual hormones inhibit the Th2 reaction and stimulate Th1 cytokines whereas **cortisol (the stress hormone) inhibits Th1 reaction and in particular IL-2 with detrimental effects on cell mediated immune responses.**

Some pro-inflammatory interleukins like IL-1, IL-6 and TNF-α stimulate ACTH secretion and also cortisol secretion with the same detrimental effect on the organism immune system responses.

IL-1, TNF-α, IFN-γ and IL-6 play a role in the thyroid function as they inhibit the iodide uptake and the release of thyroid hormones, by hindering thyreocytes growth and thyreoglobulin synthesis.

IL1- β and tumor necrosis factor (TNF) -α inhibit thyrotropin-releasing hormone (TRH) by stimulating the secretion of somatostatine. Tumor necrosis factor (TNF) also inhibits insulin like growth factor 1 (IGF-1).

Melatonin increases the effect of interleukin IL2, IL12 and interferon (IFN) gamma, inhibits cortisol (the stress hormone) and stimulates Th1 cellular immune responses.

Hematopoietic cytokines

Haematopoietic (blood producing) stem cells reside in the bone marrow and have the unique ability to give rise to all of the different mature blood cell types and tissues. All blood cells types are divided into three lineages:

- **Erythroid cells** which are the 'oxygen carrying' red blood cells.
- **Lymphocytes (white blood cells)** derived from common lymphoid progenitors cells pertaining to the adaptive immune system.
- **Myelocytes** include granulocytes, megakaryocytes and macrophages derived from common myeloid progenitor cells, and they are involved in both innate and adaptive immunity and blood clotting.

The production of hematopoietic cells is under the tight control of a group of hematopoietic cytokines like interleukins IL 3, IL 7, IL 9, IL 11, granulocyte colony-stimulating factor (GCSF), and granulocyte-macrophage colony-stimulating factor (GM-CSF).

IL-3 stimulates hematopoietic stem cells into myeloid progenitor cells. IL 7 stimulates hematopoietic stem cells into lymphoid progenitor cells. IL 9 acts as a regulator for a variety of hematopoietic cells. IL 11 stimulates platelet development in the bone marrow. GCSF and GM-CSF stimulate stem cells to produce granulocytes (neutrophils, eosinophils, and basophils) and monocytes.

Low dose cytokines which up-regulate the production of hematopoietic cells are mainly interleukin IL 3 (myeloid), IL 7 (lymphoid), granulocyte colony-stimulating factor (GCSF) and to a lesser degree also IL 9 and IL 11.

Low dose medicine and PNEI

Pyscho-neuro-endocrine-immunology (PNEI) is the study of how psychological and neurological factors on one hand and, endocrine and immune responses, on the other hand, influence each other interdependently.

The comprehension of the constant contact, communication and interdependence of these four systems, is the key for the identification of physiopatological mechanisms which lie at the heart of many if not all illnesses.

Factors like psychological-behavioural patterns, and, above all, sustained stress can change and alter the hormonal and immunological answer.

Psychological factors are the most common trigger of PNEI imbalance. Stressful states with sustain high cortisol and adrenalin levels disturb the hypothalamic-pituitary-adrenal (HPA) axis, resulting in thyroid problems and impaired immune responses.

In the PNEI vision, the neuroendocrine and immunitary systems act, respectively, as sense organs in the management of cognitive and non-cognitive stressors. Exposure to repeated cognitive, non-cognitive, physical or environmental psycho-emotional stress of sufficient intensity can cause or exacerbate an imbalance (up or down–regulation) in the formation and metabolism of cerebral chemicals like dopamine, serotonin, noradrenaline which are involved in mood regulation, attention, appetite control, reward, addiction and chronic inflammation .

As we have already seen, in low dose medicine one can use various cytokines, growth factors, hormones and neurotransmitters with the intention to up-regulate or down-regulate each and every branch of the PNEI system without any side effects, and, most important, without altering the physiological biorhythm of the individual.

Relevant terminology:

- **Cytokine**: general name for small messenger and signaling molecule (protein, glycoprotein, and peptide) released by cells which has a specific effect on the interactions between cells.
- **Interleukin:** name for a specific signaling molecule (cytokine) expressed by white blood cells and pertaining to the immune system.
- **Interferon:** cytokine or chemical substance (protein) made and released by host cells in response to the presence of pathogens such as viruses, bacteria, parasites or tumor cells, which triggers the protective defenses of the immune system to eradicate such pathogens or tumors.
- **Lymphocyte:** a type of white blood cell that plays a central role in the adaptive or acquired immune system.
- **Protein:** name for large biological molecule consisting of one or more chains of amino acids performing a vast array of functions within living organisms, including catalyzing

metabolic reactions, replicating DNA, responding to stimuli, and transporting molecules from one location to another.

- **Peptide:** name for a smaller protein-like chemical compound that is composed of a chain of two or maximum 50 amino acids and is distinguished from a protein on the basis of the smaller size. Many hormones and antibiotics are peptides.
- **Neuropeptide:** general name for a peptide (small protein) signaling molecule used by neurons to communicate with each other.
- **Neurotransmitter:** chemical substance (amino acid, peptide, or monoamine) which transmits signals between neurons and target cells of the nervous system (synapses).
- **Growth factor:** chemical substance, usually a protein or a steroid hormone, which acts as a signaling molecule, capable of stimulating cellular growth, proliferation and cellular differentiation. Growth factors play an important role in promoting cellular differentiation and cell division.
- **Neurotrophin or Neurotrophic factor:** a family of proteins that are responsible for the growth and survival of developing neurons and the maintenance of mature neurons.
- **Hormone:** a general name for a chemical messenger molecule that transports a signal from one cell to another. In humans, endocrine hormones are usually residing within a particular endocrine gland and directly released into the bloodstream.

Important note

In the following chapters under the name of some but not all specific cytokines, growth factors or hormones I have attempted to give the 'general flavour' of the molecule, but this should not confuse the reader in thinking that this is the only function of the molecule; **one should read well each complete description and indication before coming to any conclusion about each specific low dose molecule.**

I know that the medical scientist will find the decision to label each molecule reductive and maybe unacceptable and for this I apologize, but my attempt is to facilitate the general reader to deal with difficult concepts.

Chapter 3

Low dose interleukins and interferons and their main indications

The term interleukin refers to a cytokine's subgroup of signaling molecules expressed by white blood cells and pertaining to the immune system.

Interleukins are not stored within cells but are secreted rapidly, and briefly, in response to a stimulus, such as an infectious agent.

Most interleukins regulate cell growth, differentiation, and motility and are synthesized by T and B lymphocytes, as well as by monocytes, macrophages, and endothelial cells. They promote the development and differentiation of T and B lymphocytes, macrophages, natural killer (NK) and hematopoietic cells.

Interferon, another type of cytokine, is a chemical substance (protein) made and released by host cells in response to the presence of pathogens such, as viruses, bacteria, parasites or tumor cells which triggers the protective defenses of the immune system to eradicate the pathogen.

Interferons do not directly inhibit the virus's replication, but stimulate the infected cells and those nearby to produce proteins that prevent the virus from replicating within them.

Interferons also have immune-regulatory functions and increase the cellular-destruction capability of natural killer (NK) cells.

Three forms of interferons are known which have been classified into two types: type I includes the alpha (α) and beta (β) interferons, and type II which include only the gamma (γ) interferon.

Type I interferons (INF alpha and beta) can be produced by almost any cell upon stimulation by a virus; their primary function is to induce viral resistance in cells. Type II interferon (INF gamma) is secreted only by natural killer (NK) cells and T lymphocytes and has a wide variety of functions as for example to signal the immune system to respond to infectious agents or cancerous growth.

In the following list I have also included the description of interleukins IL1, IL6, IL17, IL23 which are either rarely used (IL1 and IL6) or not used at all (IL17 and IL23) in low dose medicine because of their highly inflammatory and detrimental effects on the organism.

The drug concentration for these molecules is picograms/ml properly dynamized through sequential activation which corresponds to the low dose homeopathic dilution of 4CH or 4C.

Interleukin 1 – (IL 1) 4C
Rarely used in low dose medicine

The first master inflammatory cytokine

The interleukin 1 (IL 1) family is a group of 11 cytokines, which can trigger a complex network of pro-inflammatory and endothelial cells by regulating and initiating inflammatory responses.

The most commonly used and studied cytokines of the IL-1 family are IL-1 α and IL-1β because of their role in mediating inflammatory diseases.

More than any other cytokine family, the interleukin 1 family is closely linked to the innate immune responses.

The two forms of interleukin-1, alpha and beta are made mainly by one type of white blood cell, the macrophages, and help another type of white blood cell, the lymphocytes to fight off infections; in particular they induce the production of interleukin-2 by T helper cells.

They also help leukocytes (white blood cells) to pass through blood vessel walls to the sites of infection and cause fever by affecting areas of the brain that control body temperature.

IL-1 α and IL-1β are used rarely on their own and, in any case, always for short periods of time as a biological response modifier to boost and trigger the immune system responses when these are impaired and deranged, and, especially, to induce a fever reaction.

Indications: used as an immune response starter and to induce a fever reaction in non reactive patients. General asthenia.

Anti - Interleukin 1 – (Anti IL 1) 4C

The anti-inflammatory receptor antagonist cytokine

IL-1 receptor antagonist regulates excessive production of pro-inflammatory Interleukins IL 1, IL 6 and tumor necrosis factor (TNF).

Indications: Acute inflammatory and painful conditions, especially fever; to be associated with the classic homeopathic anti-inflammatory remedies. Headaches, migraines, muscular and skeletal inflammatory conditions, brain and nervous system inflammatory conditions, cardiovascular conditions and atherosclerosis. Useful in most autoimmune diseases such as rheumatoid arthritis, thyroiditis and multiple sclerosis. It is also used to slow down cartilage degeneration in osteoarthritis and osteoarticular conditions.

Interleukin 2 – (IL 2) 4C

The 'long life' cytokine

IL 2 stimulates T and B lymphocytes and NK cells; it regulates the adaptive immune system and stimulates cell-mediated immune responses.

IL 2 is a 'master' cytokine for the discrimination between self and non-self which is a hallmark of healthy immune system. In fact, IL-2 is necessary during T cell development in the thymus for the maturation of regulatory T cells (T-reg cells).

After exiting from the thymus, T reg cells function to prevent other T cells from recognizing and reacting against self antigens, which could result in autoimmunity.

IL 2 is also pivotal for the growth, proliferation, and differentiation of T cells to become 'effector' T cells.

IL 2 is able to facilitate antibody production and response, especially immunoglobulins produced by B cells.

Also, IL2 induces the differentiation and proliferation of natural killer (NK) cells, natural killer T cells (NKT cells), and increases the production of lymphokine-activated killer cells (LAK cells), active cytotoxic cells which are able to destroy tumor cells that were already known to be resistant to NK cells activity.

The production of IL 2 decreases with age (along with the hormone melatonin and the growth factor IGF-1) which is one of the reasons why elderly people are more susceptible to infections and cancer.

Indications: all immunodeficiency conditions, aging, chronic viral and bacterial infections, colds and flu, adjuvant in cancer therapy and during chemotherapy. Support for HIV and AIDS therapy. Burning sensation in the mouth, stomatitis and mouth ulcers.

Interleukin 3 – (IL 3)

The hematopoietic cytokine

IL-3 stimulates the hematopoietic stem cells into myeloid progenitor cells.
IL 3 is secreted by basophils and activated T cells to support growth and differentiation of T cells from the bone marrow.
It works with the colony stimulating factors to stimulate progenitor cells in the bone marrow to mature and mobilize.
It is capable of supporting the proliferation of a broad range of hematopoietic cell types and it is involved in a variety of cell activities such as cell growth, differentiation and apoptosis.
IL 3 inhibits osteoclast formation, bone resorption and collagen degradation.
IL 3 has been shown to also possess neurotrophic activity, and it may be associated with neurologic disorders.

Indications: hematopoietic disorders, neutropenia during and post chemotherapy and radiotherapy. Also indicated during antiviral therapies, parasitic infections, tonsillitis and aplastic anemia. Support treatment in osteoporosis.

Interleukin 4 – (IL 4) 4C

The anti-inflammatory cytokine

IL 4 is the main cytokine to induce differentiation of naive T helper cells into T helper 2 (Th2) cells which, upon activation, subsequently produce additional IL-4.
IL 4 is important in generating protective immunity against all parasitic infections. It stimulates the proliferation of B lymphocytes and mast cells and induces a B-cell class switching to IgE antibodies.

IL-4 directs bone marrow progenitor cells to differentiate into Th2 cytokine-producing eosinophils. It is antagonist to the production of Th1 cells, macrophages, IFN-gamma, and IL-12. It also inhibits cell activation of NK cells induced by IL2.

IL4 is important in the treatment of inflammatory diseases and autoimmune diseases since it inhibits the production and proliferation of inflammatory cytokines such as IL1, IL6 and TNF alpha by monocytes and by T-cells.

IL 4 also helps the immune system to deal with environmental and industrial toxins and plays a critical role in the higher functions of the brain, such as memory and learning.

IL4 is involved in the pathogenesis of chronic lymphocytic leukemia disease by preventing both the death and the proliferation of the malignant B-cells.

IL-4 is the key inducer of all allergic reactions.

Indications: all autoimmune diseases like diabetes type 1, rheumatoid arthritis and multiple sclerosis. Chronic inflammatory diseases. Wound repair. Mental fatigue. Useful in the detoxification from pollutants. Mycosis (fungal infections).

Interleukin 5 – (IL 5) 4C

IL 5 is produced by T helper 2 (Th2) cells and mast cells.

IL-5 stimulates B cell growth and plays a major role in the regulation of eosinophil formation, maturation, recruitment and survival, therefore it has s a pivotal role in innate and acquired immune responses.

IL 5 over production is associated with eosinophilia and with a wide variety of conditions, including asthma and atopic diseases, helminth infections, drug hypersensitivity and neoplastic diseases such as Hodgkin and, to a lesser degree, non-Hodgkin lymphoma and leukemia.

Indications: parasitic infections, constipation and flatulence, abdominal cramp-like pains.

Interleukin 6 – (IL 6) 4C
Rarely used in low dose medicine

The most important inflammatory cytokine

IL 6 is produced by T lymphocytes, monocytes, endothelial cells, fibroblasts and neoplastic cells and its target cells are B lymphocytes and hepatocytes.

IL-6 is an important mediator of fever during the acute phase response, and plays a key role (with IL 1) in acute and chronic inflammation.

IL-6 acts to stimulate immune responses during infection and after trauma, especially burns or other tissue damage leading to inflammation.

In epithelial, endothelial and fibroblasts cells the secretion of IL6 is induced by IL 17.

IL-6 also activates the hypothalamus-pituitary (HPA) axis and as a consequence the stress hormone cortisol.

IL-6 is also considered a 'myokine', a cytokine produced from muscle, and it is elevated in response to muscle contraction during exercise, which precedes the appearance of other cytokines in the circulation.

The overproduction of IL 6 has been observed in various inflammatory and auto-immune pathological conditions such as rheumatoid arthritis, multiple myeloma, Castleman's disease, chronic polyarthritis, Crohn's disease, diabetes, atherosclerosis, depression, Alzheimer's disease, systemic lupus erythematosus (SLE), prostate cancer, Behçet's disease and liver cirrhosis.

The induction of epigenetic modification by IL-6 has been proposed as a mechanism in the pathology of schizophrenia and depression, and the effects of IL-6 on depression are mediated through the repression of brain-derived neurotrophic factor (BDNF) in the brain.

IL 6 synthesis is inhibited by Anti –IL1, IL-4, IFN-gamma, and leukotrienes.

Indications: It can be useful for very short periods in order to provoke an inflammatory response and activation of B and T cells in case of recurrent bacterial infections and immune deficiency.

Interleukin 7 – (IL 7) 4C

An immune system support cytokine

IL 7 stimulates the hematopoietic stem cells into lymphoid progenitor cells and the proliferation of all cells in the lymphoid lineage such as B cells, T cells and NK cells and in particular it stimulates the antitumoral action of cytotoxic T lymphocytes.

Since it acts as a lymphocytes growth factor it is of particular importance for B and T cell survival and development.

IL7 is critical for immune homeostasis and it could also be beneficial in improving immune recovery after stem cell transplant.

IL7 has been shown to induce LAK (lymphokine-activated killer) cells activity comparable quantitatively to that induced by IL2, moreover, IL-7 increases the immunological effect of IL-2 by 5 times.

Indications: immunodeficiency conditions such as AIDS, recurrent viral infections, HIV, adjuvant therapy for cancer and during chemotherapy. Also useful in wound repair.

Interleukin 8 – (IL 8) 4C

Important inflammatory cytokine

IL-8 is a chemokine produced by stimulated monocytes, epithelial cells, endothelial cells, fibroblasts, and macrophages.

The synthesis of IL8 is strongly stimulated by IL1 and TNF-alpha and therefore is implicated in a number of inflammatory responses at different levels and interplay.

In epithelial, endothelial, and fibroblastic cells, the secretion of IL8 is induced by IL1.

Glucocorticoids, IL4, TGF-beta and **vitamin D3 inhibit the synthesis of IL8.**

IL-8 is believed to play a role in the pathogenesis of bronchiolitis, a common respiratory disease caused by viral infection and is also a strong promoter of angiogenesis and tumor growth.

Other common ailments believed to be promoted by high levels of IL8 are: gastrointestinal inflammatory pathologies, rheumatoid arthritis (RA), psoriasis and septic syndromes.

Indications: recurrent bacterial infections.

Interleukin 9 – (IL 9) 4C

IL 9 is produced by T lymphocytes, especially T helper 2 (Th2) cells of adaptive immunity.

IL-9, in synergy with IL-4, mediates IgE and IgG antibody production from human B cells without having any effect on IgM production, and also stimulates mast cells production.

Along with IL-2 it stimulates the proliferation of T cells, and with IL3 can enhance hematopoiesis.

Th17 cells, which are defined by secretion of IL-17, may also secrete IL-9, but in contrast, IL 23, a cytokine required for maintenance of the IL-17 secretion, has inhibitory effects on IL-9 production.

TGF-β and IL-4 are the most potent cytokines in promoting the generation of IL-9 secreting cells, although also regulatory T cells (Treg) may produce IL-9.

In contrast with IL-2 and IL 25 which promote its production, IFN-γ inhibits IL-9 production.

A very recent study demonstrated that IL-9 substantially inhibits melanoma growth as well as lung carcinoma growth and provides a protective role in immunity to intestinal parasites.

IL-9 demonstrates pro-inflammatory activity in allergic inflammation that is at least partially dependent on the presence of other Th2 cytokines, and can also play a role in the development of acute myeloblastic leukemia.

Indications: melanoma, lung carcinoma, asthenia, adjuvant and supportive during vaccinations, erythroid proliferation disorders, water retention.

Interleukin 10 – (IL 10) 4C

The master anti-inflammatory cytokine

IL 10 is primarily produced by monocytes, macrophages, T helper 2 (Th2) lymphocytes, regulatory T cells, and by a certain subset of activated T and B cells.

IL10 regulates the reactivity of the organism and inhibits the synthesis of most pro- inflammatory cytokines such as IL1, IL6, IL8, IL12, IL23 and tumor necrosis factor (TNF) and also the Th1 sub populations of T-cells such as IFN-gamma and IL2.

IL 10 regulates cell cycles and prevents nitric oxides and oxidative stress, it suppresses metastasis and tumor invasion.

Since it inhibits the release of IL 1 and TNF it is able to slow down cartilage erosion.

IL-10 can stimulate the synthesis of IgE antibodies and acts synergically with IL 4 to inhibit cell mediated immunity. **It also prevents insulin resistance and insulin sensitivity.**

Indications: regulation and modulation of the immunotolerance processes and all chronic inflammatory responses. Useful in most autoimmune diseases, diabetes mellitus type I and II, rheumatoid arthritis, septic shock, Crohn's disease, psoriasis, transplantation rejection. Cartilage protection in all auto immune conditions and all chronic inflammatory conditions. Chronic pain syndromes, itching with a burning sensation.

Interleukin 11 – (IL 11) 4C

IL-11 has been demonstrated to improve platelet recovery after chemotherapy-induced thrombocytopenia, it acts to attenuate the production of pro-inflammatory cytokines, it modulates antigen-antibody responses, and it participates in the regulation of bone cell proliferation and differentiation, and it may be useful as an alternative therapy for osteoporosis.

IL-11 functions to control inflammation, ameliorate tissue damage, and maintain cytokine homeostasis during infection by acting on various cell types including hematopoietic precursor cells, macrophages, epithelial and T cells.

In gastrointestinal inflammation, IL-11 has been of particular interest due to its anti-inflammatory and mucosal protective effects.

IL-11 treatment significantly reduces chemotherapy related morbidity and mortality and it is associated with accelerated recovery of both hematopoiesis and the immune response during chemotherapy. IL 11 also increases platelet formation and is involved in bone formation.

Indications: gastric acidity, hematopoietic conditions, skin eruptions, specific infections and inflammatory conditions, bone healing with PTH (see low dose hormones), basic regulation during immunotherapy.

Interleukin 12 – (IL 12) 4C

The cancer support cytokine

IL 12 is produced by activated phagocytic cells such as monocytes, macrophages, neutrophils and by dendritic cells upon stimulation by bacteria, viruses, and parasites.

IL 12 is also known as a T cell-stimulating factor because it can stimulate the growth and function of T cells and especially the differentiation of naive T cells into Th1 cells (cell mediated immunity).

IL-12 enhances the cytotoxic activity of NK cells and CD8+ cytotoxic T lymphocytes and also induces the synthesis of IFN-gamma, IL2, and TNF-alpha (TNF-α).

IL-12 inhibits the synthesis of IgE induced by IL-4 and can therefore be useful in allergic diseases.

IL 12 has anti-angiogenic (it can block the formation of new blood vessels), anti-tumoral and anti-metastatic activity, and because of this, it has been proposed by immunologists as a possible anti-cancer drug (although in pharmacological doses it can cause many side-effects).

IL 12 is the most important cytokine with IL 2 and interferon gamma (IFN-gamma) in neoplastic pathologies (cancer support therapy) in general and especially melanomas and kidneys carcinoma.

IL 12 has been proved to be up-regulated in some auto-immune diseases like multiple sclerosis (MS) and diabetes type 1.

Indications: neoplastic diseases (tumors), all immunodeficiency conditions such as AIDS, HIV and recurrent viral and bacterial infections. Recurring cough, nasal obstruction, itching and parossistic sneezing. Useful in the prevention of allergic manifestations, allergic rhinitis, hyper-lacrimation, edemas, skin reddening, hypersensitivity and dermatitis.

Interleukin 17 family – (IL 17 and 17 A/B/C/D/E/F) Not used in low dose medicine

The auto-immunity inducing cytokine

IL 17 functions as a pro-inflammatory cytokine that responds to extracellular pathogens and induces destruction of the pathogen's cellular matrix.

IL 17 acts synergistically with tumor necrosis factor (TNF) and IL 1 to induce the production of many other **pro-inflammatory** cytokines such as IL-6, G-CSF, GM-CSF, IL-1β, TNF-α, IL-8, and prostaglandins from many cell types (fibroblasts, endothelial cells, epithelial cells, and macrophages).

IL-17 is also essential to a subset of T-Cells called T helper 17 (Th17) lymphocytes which have been linked to many immune/autoimmune related diseases including rheumatoid arthritis (RA), allergic responses and asthma, systemic lupus erythematosus (SLE), and psoriasis.

Interleukin 23 – (IL 23)
Not used in low dose medicine

The auto-immunity inducing cytokine

IL-23 induces the differentiation of naive CD4+T cells into a highly pathogenic subset of T helper cells (Th17) that produce pro –inflammatory cytokines IL-17, IL-17F, IL-6, and TNF-alpha. In conjunction with IL-6 and TGF-β1, IL 23 stimulates naive CD4+ T cells to differentiate into a novel subset of cells called Th17 cells, which are distinct from the classical Th1 cells and Th2 cells cells.

Th17 cells produce IL 17, a pro-inflammatory cytokine that enhances T cell priming and stimulates the production of other pro-inflammatory cytokines such as IL-1, IL-6 and TNF-alpha resulting in chronic inflammation.

Moreover, IL23 has been shown to stimulate the production of IFN- γ by PHA blast T-cells and memory T-cells.

As we have already seen, Th17 lymphocytes have been linked to many immune/autoimmune related diseases including rheumatoid arthritis (RA), allergic responses and asthma, systemic lupus erythematosus (SLE), and psoriasis.

Interferons

Interferons are proteins which possess antiviral, antimicrobic, antiproliferative and immunomodulating properties and play an important role in the first line of defense against pathogens such as viruses, bacteria, parasites or tumor cells; interferons are also able to influence the metabolism and the growth and differentiation of cells in many different ways.

The name interferon refers to their ability to 'interfere' with the viral replication within host cells.

One should bear in mind that interferons don't have a direct action on viruses, but they are important mediators of early defense against infections which inform the nearby cells to prepare their antiviral defenses in order to block the infection and damage.

Interferons have also many other functions such as to activate immune cells, like natural killer (NK) and natural killer T (NKT) cells and macrophages, increase recognition of infected or tumor cells by up-regulating antigen presentation to T lymphocytes and to increase the ability of uninfected cells to resist new infection by virus.

Many viruses have evolved mechanisms to resist interferon activity, by preventing further interferon production, and by inhibiting the functions of proteins that are induced by interferons.

Some of the viruses able to inhibit interferon signaling include: Japanese Encephalitis Virus (JEV), dengue type 2 and viruses of the herpes family, such as cytomegalovirus (HCMV) and Kaposi's sarcoma herpesvirus (KSHV or HHV8).

Interferons are usually classified into two main types: type 1 which includes two interferons such as IFN α and IFN β and type 2 which includes only IFN γ.

Interferon alpha – (INF α) – 4C

The 'anti viral' cytokine

IFN-α is involved in both the innate and adaptive immune response and it is produced by virus infected cells, mainly monocytes and macrophages.

IFN-α antiviral effect is expressed by activation of macrophages, natural killers (NK) cells, T helper (Th) lymphocytes, cytotoxic (CD8 +) T lymphocytes and also the synthesis of the major histocompatibility complex (MHC).

IFN-α activity in the early phase of immune response is synergic with other cytokines such as IL 2.

The growth of some tumor cell types is inhibited by IFN-alpha which may stimulate also the synthesis of tumor-associated cell surface antigens.

In renal carcinomas IFN-alpha reduces the expression of receptors for epidermal growth factor (EGF) and also inhibits the growth of fibroblasts and monocytes in vitro.

IFN-alpha also inhibits the proliferation of B-cells and selectively blocks the expression of some mitochondrial genes.

Indications: Recurrent and acute viral infections especially in the initial response. Antiproliferative effects, useful in cancer support therapy.

Interferon beta – (INF β) – 4C

IFN-beta is produced mainly by fibroblasts and some epithelial cell types, by viruses and other micro-organisms and also by some cytokines such as tumor necrosis factor (TNF) and IL1.

IFN-beta is involved in the regulation of non specific humoral immune responses and immune responses against viral infections; it stimulates the activity of T reg cells by reducing the production of pro-inflammatory cytokines.

IFN-beta balances the expression of pro-and anti-inflammatory agents in the brain, and reduces the number of inflammatory cells that cross the blood brain barrier.

Overall, therapy with interferon beta leads to a reduction of neuron inflammation; moreover, it is also thought to increase the production of nerve growth factor (NGF) and consequently improve neuronal survival.

IFN-beta tends to prevent disease activity in patients with multiple sclerosis (MS) and it has been used combination with IFN-alpha in the treatment of chronic active hepatitis B.

Indications: support treatment for multiple sclerosis (MS).

Interferon gamma – (INF γ) – 4C

The immune system support cytokine

IFN- γ is produced mainly by T-cells, natural killer T (NKT) cells and natural killer (NK) cells in response to antigenic (virus, bacteria, parasites) and mitogenic (cell division) stimulation.

IFN-γ has anti-viral, anti-microbic and anti-tumoral effects, but it is also able to potentiate the effects of the type I interferons such as IFN-α and IFN- β and to stimulate macrophages to kill bacteria that have been previously engulfed.

IFN-gamma can be used to treat intra-cellular persistent infections within macrophages such as toxoplasmosis, leishmaniasis, mycobacteriosis.

IFN-gamma released by Th1 cells is also important in regulating and counteracting the Th2 driven allergic response.

IFN-γ secretion is stimulated by IL-2, IL-12 and IL-18 and it is inhibited by IL-4, IL-10, TGF-β and glucocorticoids.

Indications: Antiproliferative effects, useful in cancer therapy. Antiviral and highly antibacterial activity especially during the initial onset of infections. Opportunistic infections in immune compromised patients. Cold and flu prevention and therapy. Allergic syndromes prevention and cure.

Tumor necrosis factor – TNF α – 4C

An important inflammatory cytokine

TNF is a member of a group of cytokines that stimulate the acute phase reaction and is secreted mainly by macrophages, monocytes, neutrophils, T-cells, NK-cells and neurons following their stimulation by bacteria.

TNF-alpha has a wide spectrum of biological activities, generally together with IL-1 and IL-6, such as prostaglandin synthesis by hypothalamic cells, HPA (hypothalamic-pituitary-adrenal) axis stimulation by stimulating the release of corticotropin releasing hormone (CRH), appetite suppression, fever induction, hepatocytes stimulation for the production of acute phase proteins, hypoglycemia, insulin resistance and stimulation of phagocytosis on macrophages.

High concentrations of TNF induce shock-like symptoms whereas the prolonged exposure to low concentrations of TNF can result in cachexia.

Indications: complementary therapy for tumours, chronic bacterial infections, recurrent colds and immune system hypo reactivity in general, appetite control and suppression.

Interleukins and interferons regulation chart

Interleukin	Up-regulation	Down-regulation
IL 1	IL 1 -4C	Anti IL1/IL 10-4C
IL 2	IL 2 -4C	IL 4-4C/ IL 11-4C
IL 3	IL 3-4C	IL 10-4C
IL 4	IL 4-4C	INF γ-4C/ IL 12-4C
IL 5	IL 5-4C	TGF β-4C
IL 6	IL 6-4C	Anti IL1/IL 10-4C/ IL 4-4C
IL 7	IL 7-4C	TGF β-4C / IL 10-4C
IL 8	IL 8-4C	TGF β-4C / IL 10-4C
IL 9	IL 9-4C	IL 10-4C
IL 10	IL 10-4C	IL 1 -4C/ IL 6-4C TNF-4C/ IL 10-4C
IL 11	IL 11-4C	IL 2 -4C
IL 12	IL 12-4C	IL 4-4C/ IL 10-4C
IL 13	IL 13-4C	INF γ-4C/ IL 12-4C
IL17	IL 23/IL 6	IL 4-4C /INF γ-4C
IL 23	IL 23/IL 17/ IL 6	IL 4-4C /INF γ-4C
INF α -β -γ	INF α -β -γ-4C	IL 4-4C/ IL 10-4C
TNF	TNF-4C	Anti IL1/IL 10-4C

Chapter 4

Low dose growth factors and their main indications

Growth factors are hormone- like chemical molecules, sometimes small proteins, which acts as signaling molecules and are capable of stimulating cellular growth, proliferation and cellular differentiation.

Growth factors play an important role in promoting cellular differentiation and cell division, and the abnormal production and regulation of growth factors can play a role in the progression of several diseases.

Some growth factors are similar to hormones in that they can be secreted into the blood stream, which carries them to their target tissues, however, **whereas the production of hormones is limited to glandular tissue, growth factors can be produced by many different types of tissue.**

The drug concentration for these molecules is picograms/ml properly dynamized through sequential activation which corresponds to the low dose homeopathic dilution of 4CH or 4C.

Epidermal growth factor – EGF – 4C

Epidermal Growth Factor (EGF) is a small protein that stimulates cell growth, proliferation, and differentiation.

EGF is a small polypeptide which is distributed throughout a wide number of tissues and body fluid and it can generally be found in human platelets, macrophages, urine, saliva, milk, and plasma.

Salivary EGF plays an important physiological role in the maintenance of esophageal and gastric tissue integrity. The biological effects of salivary EGF includes healing of oral and gastro-esophageal ulcers, inhibition of gastric acid secretion, stimulation of DNA synthesis as well as mucosal protection from factors such as gastric acid, bile acids, pepsin, and trypsin and to physical, chemical and bacterial agents.

The production of EGF has been shown to be stimulated by testosterone and to be inhibited by estrogens.

In the central nervous system EGF influences the activity of some types of GABA and dopaminergic neurons.

In several cell types EGF down regulates the expression of the receptor for TGF-beta.

EGF stimulates blood flow and circulation and may prevent fibrosis. EGF alone or in combination with other cytokines such as FGF is an important factor in mediating wound healing processes and skin repair.

Indications: It is very useful in gastric hyperacidity, ulcerative gastritis and epigastric fullness with pain. Ophthalmic conditions including optic nerve conditions and blurred vision with presence of light spots. since low dose EGF stimulates epithelial cells, endothelial cells and fibroblasts, it can be used in aesthetic treatment applications mixed with a neutral cream to rejuvenate and regenerate skin, repair sun damage, to repair wounds, especially lacerations and burns, itchy and chapped skin.

Since it stimulates angiogenesis is contraindicated during cancer treatments.

Fibroblast growth factor – FGF-1 – 4C

Fibroblast growth factors, (FGF) are a family of multifunctional proteins which play an important role in the processes of proliferation and differentiation of a wide variety of cells and tissues.

The fibroblast growth factors family is mainly involved in developmental processes and new growth of blood vessels, fibroblasts and endothelial cells, mesoderm induction, neural induction and neural development.

In mature tissues FGF stimulates angiogenesis, new growth of blood vessels, keratinocyte, fibroblasts and endothelial cells, and wound healing processes.

Indications: wound healing, anti age therapy, metabolic syndrome, hyperlipidemia and insulin resistance, cardiovascular conditions. Anti-inflammatory effect on muscle and bones, osteoarthritis, joints and cartilage repair.
Since it stimulates angiogenesis is contraindicated during cancer treatments.

Granulocyte colony stimulating factor – GCSF – 4C

The immune system starter cytokine

Granulocyte colony-stimulating factor (G-CSF or GCSF) is a glycoprotein which stimulates the proliferation and differentiation of hematopoietic progenitor cells from the bone marrow into granulocytes (white blood cells) and neutrophils.

G-CSF is produced by monocytes, macrophages, and neutrophils after cell activation and it is also produced by stromal cells, fibroblasts, and endothelial cells.

G-CSF triggers the reactivity and raises the sensitivity of the immune system, and it enhances the antibody-dependent cell mediated cytotoxicity of granulocytes against tumor cells.

Indications: neutropenia during and post chemotherapy. Supportive treatment during transplant and leukemia. Useful in the initial phase of all treatments especially during bacterial, viral and fungal infections (mycosis) and fever.

Insulin-like growth factor 1 – IGF 1– 4C

The 'anti age' growth factor

Insulin-like growth factor 1 (IGF-1), is a protein similar in molecular structure to insulin mainly produced by the liver.

Its production is stimulated by the growth hormone (GH) and can be retarded by under nutrition or malnutrition, growth hormone insensitivity, lack of growth hormone receptors and it is also reduced with age.

In children, it stimulates bone growth and development of organs such as the heart, liver, and kidneys.

In humans, the growth hormone (GH) made in the anterior pituitary gland stimulates the liver to produce insulin-like growth factor 1 (IGF-1) which then stimulates and has a growth-promoting effect on almost every cell in the body, especially kidney, muscles, cartilage, liver, nerves, skin, hematopoietic cells, and lungs.

Since IGF-1 has been demonstrated to stimulate proteoglycans and collagen synthesis, it plays an important role in osteoarthritis and cartilage homeostasis. Low levels of IGF-1 can induce chronic endocrine conditions.

Indications: general growth disorders, growth and maintenance of nerve tissue and cartilage repair, osteoarthritis. Metabolic syndrome, insulin resistance, obesity and high cholesterol levels, liver steatosis (fatty liver), enlarged spleen, diabetic neuropathy, support treatment during menopause (IGF levels decrease). Fibromyalgia, in combination with IL 10, Anti IL 1 and β Endorphin. Anti age therapy and UV protection. Contraindicated in prostate cancer.

Transforming growth factor beta – TGF β – 4C

The anti-inflammatory and tissue repair cytokine

Transforming growth factor beta (TGF-β) is a protein which controls proliferation, cellular differentiation, and other functions in most cells.

TGF-beta is secreted by many cell types, including macrophages and Th2 and Th3 lymphocytes.

TGF-beta stimulates fibroblast proliferation, angiogenesis (especially in connective tissue) and therefore **is involved in different stages of healing and connective tissue regeneration with powerful regulating action on inflammatory events.**

Indications: chronic inflammation and pain syndromes, tendon, ligament and muscle repair. Connective tissue regeneration, musculoskeletal neuropathies.

Growth factors/interleukins regulation chart

Growth factor	Up-regulation	Down-regulation
GCSF	GCSF -4C	IL 4-4C/ IL 10-4C
TGF β	TGF β-4C	IL 12-4C/ IL 5-4C/ IL 7-4C/ IL 8-4C

Chapter 5

Low dose neurotrophic factors and their main indications

Neurotrophins or neurotrophic factors are a family of proteins that are responsible for the growth and survival of developing neurons and the maintenance of mature neurons.

Neurotrophic factors promote the initial growth and development of neurons in the central nervous system and peripheral nervous system and they are capable of re-growing damaged neurons.

They also induce differentiation of progenitor cells to form new neurons. Neurotrophins can generally be subdivided into five structurally related types: Nerve Growth Factor (NGF), Brain-Derived Neurotrophic Factor (BDNF), Ciliary Neurothrophic Factor (CNTF), Neurotrophin-3 (NT-3) and Neurotrophin-4 (NT-4).

The drug concentration for these molecules is picograms/ml properly dynamized through sequential activation which corresponds to the low dose homeopathic dilution of 4CH or 4C.

Nerve Growth Factor (NGF) – 4C

The nerve regenerative and repairing neurotrophine

NGF was the first neurotrophic factor to be discovered by Professors Rita Levi-Montalcini and Stanley Cohen in the 1950s; however, its discovery, along with the discovery of other neurotrophins, was not widely recognized until 1986.

NGF is synthesized in the hypothalamus, pituitary, thyroid gland, testis, and it is also produced by vascular smooth muscle cells and fibroblasts.

The expression of NGF in specific neurons of the central nervous system (cortex, hippocampus) can be influenced positively by glutamate and negatively by GABA stimulating neuronal activity.

NGF stimulates the growth and differentiation of B-cells and the growth of T-cells and also promotes the proliferation of mast cells.

Vitamin D3 is potent inducer of NGF synthesis (a possible reason for vitamin D antidepressant action), while glucocorticoids are potent NGF inhibitors.

Studies have shown that NGF seems to prevent or reduce neuronal degeneration in neurodegenerative diseases. It has also been shown to promote peripheral nerve regeneration and has neuroprotective effects on myelin, thus it is indicated in multiple sclerosis (MS).

NGF seems to protect cholinergic neurons in Alzheimer's disease which is characterized by a selective degeneration of these cells.

Indications: neuralgic pain and neurological damage, multiple sclerosis (MS), diabetes-associated polyneuropathies and chemotherapy induced neuropathies, Alzheimer's disease, memory and mood disorders and long term depression.

Brain Derived Neurotrophic Factor (BDNF) – 4C

The learning and memory support neurotrophine

BDNF was the second neurotrophic factor to be discovered after the Nerve Growth Factor (NGF).

In the brain, BDNF is expressed predominantly in the hippocampus, cortex, and synapses of the basal forebrain areas

where it is vital to learning, memory, and higher thinking. BDNF is also expressed in muscles.

BDNF selectively supports the survival of primary sensory neurons, retinal ganglia and the survival and differentiation of certain cholinergic and dopaminergic neurons. It also modulates neural plasticity and predisposition to behaviors.

BDNF can recover re-innervation in the mature cerebellum thus it is applicable in trauma of the central nervous system (CNS). Both BDNF and NGF express neuroprotective effects on myelin, thus they are indicated in multiple sclerosis (MS).

Exposure to stress and the stress hormone corticosterone has been shown to decrease the expression of BDNF which can lead to depression.

On the other hand, the expression of BDNF is increased by voluntary exercise, caloric restriction, intellectual stimulation, curcumin, the neurotransmitter glutamate and various antidepressants drugs.

Various studies have shown possible links between BDNF dysregulation and conditions such as bipolar disorder, schizophrenia, obsessive-compulsive disorder, autism, Huntington's disease, Rett syndrome and dementia, as well as anorexia nervosa and bulimia nervosa.

Post mortem analysis has shown lowered levels of BDNF in the brain tissues of people with Alzheimer's disease and a connection between depression and dementia has been suggested to be mediated by this neurotrophin.

BDNF is also a critical regulator of drug dependency since it causes cravings in opiate-dependent people; on the other hand BDNF has a role in maintaining long-term abstinence from alcohol in people with alcohol dependency.

Indications: neurological damage, stress, depression, insomnia, neurodegenerative diseases, Huntington's disease, Alzheimer's, Parkinson's, dementia, learning, memory and mood disorders, diabetes in the elderly and alcoholism. BDNF is not indicated in case of recurring migraines, itching and also in opiate dependency.

Ciliary Neurotrophic Factor (CNTF) – 4C

CNTF is a neurotrophin predominantly found in peripheral nerve tissues which effects the growth of parasympathetic neurons and sympathetic, sensory, and spinal motor neurons.

CNTF is a potent survival factor for neurons and oligodendrocytes, and may be relevant in reducing tissue destruction during inflammatory attacks.

Since CNTF promotes the survival of motor neurons it may be possible to use this neurotrophin in the support treatment for amyotrophic lateral sclerosis (ALS), a neurodegenerative disorder characterized by a progressive degeneration of upper and lower motor neurons in the spinal cord.

CNTF has also been shown to be expressed by cells on the bone surface, and it can act to reduce the activity of osteoblasts (the bone forming cells).

Recent studies have shown that CNTF could reduce food intake and control appetite without causing hunger or stress.

Indications: support treatment for amyotrophic lateral sclerosis (ALS), eyesight disorders, retinal degeneration, brain aging, appetite control.

Neurotrophin 3 (NT3) – 4C

NT3 is a neurotrophic factor of the NGF (Nerve Growth Factor) family found in neurons of the central nervous system.

NT3 was the third neurotrophic factor to be discovered after Nerve Growth Factor (NGF) and Brain Derived Neurotrophic Factor (BDNF).

NT-3 selectively supports the survival of neuronal cell populations, it helps to support the survival and differentiation of existing neurons, and encourages the growth and differentiation of new neurons and synapses.

Indications: modulation of depression and neuronal protection during and after chemotherapy. Regulation of peripheral sensory neurons. Biological action similar to NT 4 and BDNF.

Neurotrophin 4 (NT4) – 4C

NT4 is a neurotrophic factor in the NGF (Nerve Growth Factor) family of neurotrophins.

NT 4 has a similar biological activity as NT3 and BDNF, although NT4 supports more sensory neurons than BDNF.

Indications: useful in the modulation of anxiety and in cutaneous conditions of nervous origin like psoriasis, eczema and dermatitis.

Chapter 6

Low dose hormones and neuropeptides and their main indications

The term hormone is a general name for a type of messenger molecule that transports a signal from one cell to another.

Endocrine hormones are secreted (released) directly into the bloodstream via the capillaries. They are typically specialized cells residing within a particular endocrine gland, such as the pituitary gland, the thyroid, parathyroid, pancreas, pineal gland, ovaries, and testes.

A neuropeptide is a protein-like signaling molecules (peptide) used by neurons to communicate with each other. **In some cases peptides can function in the periphery as hormones and also have neuronal functions as neuropeptides.**

Different neuropeptides are involved in a wide range of brain functions, including analgesia, reward, food intake, metabolism, reproduction, social behaviors, learning and memory.

In general, though, neuropeptides are secreted from neuronal cells (primarily neurons) and signal to neighboring cells (primarily neurons). In contrast, peptide hormones are secreted from neuroendocrine cells and travel through the blood to distant tissues where they evoke a response.

Many neuropeptides are co-released with other small-molecules called neurotransmitters, and, the term neurotransmitter is sometimes used interchangeably with the term neuropeptide.

When a neurotransmitter is released from the first neuron, it floats into the space (the synapse) between the two neurons, and it is then received by a receptor on the other side of the brain which then sends a signal down to the receiving neuron.

The drug concentration for these molecules is nanograms/ml properly dynamized through sequential activation which corresponds to the low dose homeopathic dilution of 6X or 6D.

Adrenocorticotropic hormone – (ACTH) 6X

ACTH also known as corticotropin, is a trophic hormone produced and secreted by the anterior pituitary gland.

It is an important component of the hypothalamic-pituitary-adrenal (HPA) axis and it is produced in response to corticotropin-releasing hormone (CRH) from the hypothalamus which is often secreted in response to many types of stress.

Within the pituitary gland, ACTH is produced in a process that also generates several other hormones and it stimulates the production of corticosteroids hormones such as hydrocortisone, corticosterone, cortisol, aldosterone and the sex hormones.

ACTH (and CRH) deficiency is the cause of secondary and tertiary adrenal insufficiency. In Cushing's disease, on the other hand the levels of ACTH are usually elevated.

Indications: secondary and tertiary adrenal insufficiency, memory and learning deficiency, lack of motivation, asthenia, aging, chronic stress, lack of appetite, improvement of mental performance, increase of visual alertness.

β-Endorphin 6X or 4C

The pain management hormone

Beta endorphin is a neurotransmitter found in the neurons of both the central and peripheral nervous system.

In the peripheral nervous system (PNS), beta-endorphin produce analgesia by binding to opioid receptors (particularly of the 'mu' subtype) at both pre- and post- synaptic nerve terminals, primarily exerting their effect through pre-synaptic binding.

In the central nervous system (CNS), beta-endorphin similarly binds 'mu' opioid receptors and exerts its primary action at pre-synaptic nerve terminals. However, instead of inhibiting substance P, it exerts its analgesic effect by inhibiting the release of GABA, an inhibitory neurotransmitter (see GABA section), resulting in increased production of dopamine which is associated with pleasure.

β-endorphin has approximately 80 times the analgesic potency of morphine and it is used as an analgesic by the body to numb pain during traumas. That is the reason why humans start to feel better immediately after an acute trauma even though the symptoms are fully present. For the reasons mentioned above, β-endorphin is also believed to have a number of other benefits including promoting a feeling of well-being and increasing relaxation.

Indications: modulation of inflammatory pain, acute and chronic pain management.

β - Estradiol 6X

Estradiol is a sex hormone and the major estrogen in humans. **Estradiol is derived from cholesterol and has a critical impact on reproductive and sexual functioning, and also affects other organs including the bones.**

In females, during the reproductive years, most estradiol is produced by the granulosa cells of the ovaries by the aromatization of androstenedione to estrone, which is then converted to estradiol. Smaller amounts of estradiol are also produced by the adrenal cortex, by the testis, in the brain and in arterial walls.

Estradiol acts as a growth hormone for the tissue of the reproductive organs, supporting the lining of the vagina, the cervical glands, the endometrium, and the lining of the fallopian tubes.

Estradiol enhances development of secondary sex characteristics in women and it is responsible for changes in the body shape, affecting bones, joints, fat deposition, fat structure and skin composition. **In conjunction with progesterone, it prepares the endometrium for implantation.**

During the menstrual cycle, estradiol produced by the growing follicle triggers the luteinizing hormone (LH), inducing ovulation.

The production of estradiol declines after menopause which is why women after menopause experience an accelerated loss of bone mass due to a relative estrogen deficiency affecting the bones.

Indications: estrogen deficiency, menopause, hot flushes, preservation of pregnancy, breast feeding maintenance and preparation for the menstrual cycle.

Calcitonin 6X

The bone healing hormone

Calcitonin is a hormone secreted by the thyroid gland which helps to regulate calcium levels in the body.

Calcitonin decreases serum calcium concentrations by inhibiting the activity of the osteoclasts (cells responsible for the dissolution and absorption of bones) in bone tissue and by increasing calcium excretion in the urine.

It also protects against calcium loss from the skeleton during periods of calcium mobilization, such as pregnancy and, especially, lactation.

Calcitonin acts both directly on osteoclasts, resulting in inhibition of bone resorption and directly on chondrocytes, attenuating cartilage degradation and stimulating cartilage formation.

Calcitonin is often used in women with postmenopausal osteoporosis to help reduce bone loss and recently in the treatment of osteoarthritis.

Indications: osteoporosis, Paget's disease, osteoarthritis, bone loss and bone pain, hypertension.

Dopamine 6X or 4C

The reward, pleasure and satisfaction neurotransmitter

Dopamine is the neurotransmitter responsible for the reward-driven learning, motivation, healthy assertiveness, sexual arousal, emotional responses and proper immune and autonomic nervous system functions.
An increase in dopamine release in the nucleus accumbens occurs in response to a feeling of reward (like winning money, handling banknotes or making a discovery etc), sexual stimulation, feeling in love, music, and during the course of drug addiction.

There is a close association between the dopaminergic reward system and opiates, in fact, all drugs, from cocaine, heroin and nicotine to MDMA increase dopamine levels in the nucleus accumbens area of the brain, and many people like to describe a spike in dopamine as kind of feeling of 'motivation' or 'pleasure'.

In general, opioids in the central nervous system (CNS) exert their analgesic effect by increasing dopamine release and inhibiting GABA's effect on dopaminergic neurons which are those of the 'reward center'. Dopamine can also increase in the nucleus accumbens in people with post-traumatic stress disorder when they are experiencing heightened vigilance and paranoia.

In one recent study, meditation and Yoga was reported to increase the release of dopamine.

Several important diseases of the nervous system like Parkinson's disease, which is caused by loss of dopamine-secreting neurons in the substantia nigra; attention deficit hyperactivity disorder (ADHD) and restless legs syndrome (RLS) are associated with dysfunctions of the dopamine system.

Schizophrenia has been shown to involve elevated levels of dopamine activity in the mesolimbic pathway.

Dopamine cannot cross the blood-brain barrier to directly affect the central nervous system, so it cannot be given as a drug in general, but, as we have seen, **the low dose active preparation will stimulate its production physiologically when this is needed.**

Indications: mental stress, mood disorders and depression, decreased sexual arousal and lack of sexual desire, chronic fatigue syndrome and supporting treatment in Parkinson's disease. Support treatment for addictions and drug abuse.

DHEA – (Dehydroepiandrosterone) 6X

The anti-stress hormone

DHEA is an important steroid hormone produced by the adrenal glands, the gonads, and the brain.

DHEA functions as a metabolic intermediate in the biosynthesis of the male and female androgen and estrogen sex hormones. It is also an important regulator of the thyroid and pituitary glands and also has a variety of other potential biological effects.

DHEA is considered to buffer stress and the negative impact it can have on both mental and physical functions; it is a good stress barometer, because when stress levels go up, DHEA levels go down.

Long-term stress can cause elevated cortisol levels and reduced DHEA levels with devastating effects on the immune

71

system with increased risk to infections, cancer, allergies and autoimmune diseases.

DHEA levels in the body begin to decrease after the age of 30, and are reported to be low in some people with anorexia, end-stage kidney disease, type 2 diabetes, AIDS, adrenal insufficiency, and in the critically ill.

DHEA levels may also be depleted by a number of drugs, including insulin, corticosteroids and opiates.

High pharmacological doses may cause aggressiveness, irritability, trouble sleeping, growth of body or facial hair on women, stop menstruation and lower the levels of HDL cholesterol, which could raise the risk of heart disease.

Regular exercise is known to increase physiological DHEA production.

Indications: all stress related conditions, mood disorders and decreased or lack of sexual desire.

Follicle stimulating hormone – (FSH) 6X

The fertility hormone

Follicle stimulating hormone (FSH) is produced by the anterior pituitary gland and in females it stimulates the maturation of ovarian follicles and the production of the hormone estradiol; in males it stimulates sperm production.

FSH regulates the development and growth of pubertal maturation and reproductive body processes.

Follicle-stimulating hormone (FSH) and Luteinizing hormone (LH) act synergistically in reproduction and are called gonadotropins because they stimulate the gonads (the testis in males, and the ovaries in females).

Indications: ovulatory stimulation, female cycle disorders, female low libido.

Luteinizing hormone – (LH) 6X

The fertility hormone

Luteinizing hormone (LH) is produced by the anterior pituitary gland and in females it triggers ovulation and stimulates the development of the corpus luteum which, in turn, produces progesterone to prepare the endometrium for a possible implantation. In males it stimulates testosterone production.

LH is necessary to maintain luteal function for the first two weeks of the menstrual cycle.

Luteinizing hormone (LH) and Follicle-stimulating hormone (FSH) act synergistically in reproduction and are called gonadotropins because they stimulate the gonads (the testis in males, and the ovaries in females).

Indications: male and female sterility, male low libido, female cycle disorders, recurrent abortion.

GABA (gamma-Aminobutyric acid) 6X or 4C

The calming and sleep inducing neurotransmitter

GABA is the master inhibitory neurotransmitter in the central nervous system where it plays a central role in regulating neuronal excitability and muscle tone.

It is estimated that close to 40% of the synapses in the human brain work with GABA and therefore have GABA receptors.

GABA acts at inhibitory synapses in the brain by binding to specific transmembrane receptors in the plasma membrane of both pre and postsynaptic neuronal processes. Neurons that produce GABA as their output are called GABAergic neurons, and have chiefly inhibitory action on receptors.

While GABA is an inhibitory transmitter in the mature brain, its actions are primarily excitatory in the developing brain.

Pharmacological drugs which increase the available amount of GABA in central nervous system (CNS) are called GABAergic drugs. Among these we find barbiturates and benzodiazepines which have a typically relaxing, anti-anxiety, and anti-convulsive effect.

Indications: anxiety, panic attacks, mood disorders, insomnia and phobias.

Melatonin 4C or 6X

The 'long life' hormone

Melatonin is a neurohormone derivative of serotonin, secreted by the pineal gland which is the most important neuroendocrine organ in the brain.

The pineal gland translates an external signal (daily and seasonal variation in light and temperature) into a specific hormonal secretion which regulates the endocrine functions.

The principal factor affecting melatonin secretion is light, which inhibits its secretion, whereas darkness has the opposite effect from light, resulting in an increase of melatonin secretion.

Alterations in circadian rhythms may cause the onset of numerous pathologies like emotional problems (serious depression), immune deficiency, psychosomatic disorders, dermatological pathologies such as psoriasis and vitiligo, problems linked with food intake (bulimia, mental anorexia), sleep disorders, problems with puberty, and possibly cancer .

Melatonin has been proved to increase REM sleep time and dream activity, and users have reported an increase in the vividness of dreams and lucid dreaming.

Besides the regulation of circadian rhythms and sleep the pineal gland hormone melatonin has been found to directly modulate catecholamine (epinephrine and norepinephrine) and cortisol (the stress hormone) levels; it controls the diurnal cycle of glucosteroids and inhibits hydrocortisone synthesis in the adrenal glands.

During stress, elevated amounts of hydrocortisone inhibit melatonin synthesis, thereby causing vascular damage, hypertension, type 2 diabetes and eventual organ failure.

Since stress hormones affect memory processing, melatonin can be regarded as a modulator and enhancer of memory functions.

In Alzheimer's disease melatonin may prevent neuronal death caused by exposure to the amyloid beta protein, a neurotoxic substance that accumulates in the brains of patients with this disorder.

Melatonin is a powerful free-radical scavenger and wide-spectrum antioxidant, twice as active as vitamin E and with a particular role in the protection of nuclear and mitochondrial DNA.

Recent research has supported the anti-aging properties of melatonin, since it neutralizes oxidative damage and may delay the neurodegenerative process of aging.

Clinical studies indicate that melatonin is an effective preventive treatment for migraines and cluster headaches. Studies have also shown that women with low levels of melatonin secretion have been found to be more prone to develop diabetes (type 2) than women with high levels.

Melatonin interacts with the immune system by stimulating cell mediated acquired immunity and the production of cytokines and it has been proven useful in fighting viral, and bacterial infections, and potentially in the treatment of cancer.

Studies suggest that people with autism spectrum disorders (ASD) may have lower than normal levels of melatonin and that melatonin supplementation decreases sleep latency and increases total sleep time.

To conclude, we can regard melatonin as a 'starter' which, depending on the gravity of the problem, is able to regulate countless fragile mechanisms which ensure a well balanced PNEI (pyscho-neuro-endocrine-immunitary) system and the maintenance of health.

Indications: anti age therapy, to achieve a strong antioxidant effect in all stress related conditions, insomnia and sleep disorders, lucid dreaming inducer, jet lag, impotence, sterility, frigidity, mood and eating disorders, autism spectrum disorders (ASD), diabetes type2, neurodegenerative diseases (ALS, Alzheimer's), migraines, cell proliferation and cancer support therapy.

Oxytocin 6X or 4C

The bonding, love and trust hormone

Oxytocin is a hormone released by the pituitary gland which also acts as a neurotransmitter in the brain. It is released during hugging, touching, and orgasm in both sexes.

In the brain, oxytocin is involved in social recognition and bonding, romantic love, maternal behavior and may be involved in the formation of trust and generosity between people.

Because of its ability to break-down social barriers, to induce feelings of optimism, increase self-esteem, and build trust, oxytocin can help to overcome social inhibitions and fears. Since oxytocin affects social distance between adult males and females, it may be responsible for romantic attraction and subsequent monogamous bonding.

Oxytocin has the ability to reduce stress since it modulates the hypothalamic-pituitary-adrenal (HPA) axis by indirectly inhibiting the release of ACTH hormone and by reducing cortisol levels (the stress hormone).

Oxytocin has proven anti-inflammatory properties by inhibiting certain cytokines and can be of help wound healing and inflammatory pain.

The inability to secrete oxytocin is linked to sociopathy, psychopathy, narcissism, inability to feel empathy and general manipulativeness.

Oxytocin is also often used to help cervical dilation before birth since it causes contractions during the second and third stages of labor.

Indications: support treatment for autism, social phobia and anxieties, decreased sexual satisfaction, female sexual ailments.

Parathyroid hormone – (PTH) 6X

Parathyroid hormone or PTH is secreted by the parathyroid gland situated behind the thyroid gland. Calcium is tightly regulated by the PTH and bone resorption, the normal destruction of bone by osteoclasts, is indirectly stimulated by PTH which binds to osteoblasts, the cells responsible for creating bone.

When calcium levels are low, PTH induces the kidneys to reabsorb calcium and magnesium from distal tubules, and to increase production of the active form of vitamin D thereby increasing intestinal absorption of calcium, and its release from the bones. **These actions lead to a re-balance of the calcium levels in the blood.**

Indications: bone repair processes, bone traumas, and bone formation, osteoporosis and low calcium levels.

Progesterone 6X

Progesterone is a steroid hormone produced by the ovaries, the adrenal glands and, during pregnancy in the placenta. It is involved in the female menstrual cycle; it supports gestation during pregnancy and embryogenesis.

Progesterone prepares the uterus for implantation, it affects the vaginal epithelium and cervical mucus, making it thick and impenetrable to sperm and also it inhibits the muscular contractions of the uterus that would probably cause the wall to reject the adhering egg.

Following a successful implantation, progesterone helps to maintain a supportive environment for the developing fetus and after a few weeks of pregnancy, the placenta takes over the progesterone production from the ovaries and substantially increases progesterone production.

During pregnancy, progesterone stimulates the development of the glands in the breasts that are responsible for milk production and a decrease in progesterone levels following delivery is one of the triggers for milk production.

If pregnancy does not occur, progesterone levels will decrease, leading to normal menstruation (progesterone-withdrawal bleeding).

Progesterone is also a neurosteroid and as such it can affect the central nervous system by affecting synaptic functioning and neuron myelination.

Since progesterone inhibits the enzyme monoamine oxidase (MAO) which is responsible for breaking down serotonin, and also enhances the serotonin receptors function in the brain, low levels of progesterone can negatively affect mood, trigger migraines and play a role in nicotine and alcohol addiction. Moreover, in the brain, progesterone binds to GABA receptors with a positive effect on anxiety and relaxation.

Indications: menstrual cycle disorders, pre-menstrual syndrome (PMS) including migraines and depression, menstrual pain and pre-menopause.

Serotonin 6X

The 'feel good' neurotransmitter

Serotonin is a neurotransmitter which plays an important role in regulating mood, memory, learning and blood pressure, as well as appetite and body temperature.

Serotonin is synthesized from tryptophan (an essential amino acid) and it is primarily found in the gastrointestinal tract (90%), where it regulates bowel movement, and in the central nervous system (CNS) where it performs its primary functions.

Serotonin is regarded as an adaptogen, since it promotes contentment and it is a responsible for the regulation of mood, appetite and normal sleep. It also has some cognitive functions, including memory and learning.

Some of the natural strategies to stimulate serotonin production are exposure to bright light, as there is a positive correlation and interaction between serotonin synthesis and bright light; exercise, which, as some research suggests, seem to increase serotonin function in the brain along with its precursor tryptophan (which seem to persists after exercise); and a diet rich in tryptophan found in most protein-based foods or supplements.

According to another study, self -induced positive moods can influence positively serotonin synthesis which in turn sustains a feeling of well being.

Progesterone inhibits the enzyme 'monoamine oxidase' (MAO) which is responsible for breaking down serotonin and enhances serotonin receptivity in the female brain.

Low serotonin levels produce insomnia and depression, aggressive behaviour, increased sensitivity to pain, migraines and are associated with obsessive-compulsive eating disorders.

Alterations in serotonin levels have also been shown to regulate bone mass, where low levels can be predictor of low bone density.

The herbal extract of St.John's wort (*Hypericum perforatum)* which is often used in the treatment of mild to moderate depression and anxiety disorders seem to be effective due to several chemicals, including hypericin, hyperforin, and flavonoids which stimulate the production of the serotonin and dopamine.

Conventional antidepressant medications which work by selectively inhibiting the reuptake of serotonin in the brain can be classified as 'selective serotonin reuptake inhibitors' (SSRIs); 'monoamine oxidase inhibitors' (MAOIs) which prevent the breakdown of monoamine neurotransmitters (including serotonin) and tricyclic antidepressants (TCAs) which inhibit the reuptake of both serotonin and norepinephrine.

Indications: all mood disorders, depression, migraines, addictions and eating disorders.

Somatostatin 6X

The master inhibitory hormone

Somatostatin is an inhibitory hormone that regulates the endocrine system and affects neurotransmission and cell proliferation and inhibition of numerous hormones.

Somatostatin is produced by the hypothalamus and some other tissues such as the pancreas and the gastrointestinal tract.

In the anterior pituitary gland it inhibits the release of both the growth hormone (GH) and the thyroid-stimulating hormone (TSH).

Somatostatin secreted by the pancreas inhibits the secretion of the other pancreatic hormones such as insulin and glucagon, and reduces the activity of gastrointestinal hormones, gastric acidity and abdominal blood.

Indications: oncology diseases, cancer support treatment, hyperthyroidism.

Thyroid-stimulating hormone – (TSH) 6X

Thyroid stimulating hormone (TSH) is produced by the anterior pituitary gland upon stimulation by thyrotropin releasing hormone (TRH) produced by the hypothalamus.

TSH main function is to stimulate the thyroid gland to secrete the hormone thyroxine (T4) which is then converted into the active hormone triiodothyronine (T3), which then stimulates and affects many physiological processes in the body including metabolism. About 80% of this conversion is in the liver and other organs, and 20% in the thyroid itself.

The concentration of thyroid hormones (T3 and T4) in the blood regulates the anterior pituitary gland release of TSH; when T3 and T4 concentrations are low, the production of TSH is increased, and, conversely, when T3 and T4 concentrations are high, TSH production is decreased, and by these processes, a feedback control system is set up to regulate the amount of thyroid hormones (T3 and T4) that are present in the blood.

Indications: thyroid stimulation, overweight tendency, obesity, short-term treatment for depression, neurasthenia, water retention and metabolic slowdown.

T3– (Triiodothyronine) 6X

T3 is an active thyroid hormone produced by the follicular cells of the thyroid gland upon stimulation by the thyroid -stimulating-hormone (TSH). T3 affects almost every physiological process in the body, including growth and development, body temperature, metabolism and heart rate.

Since iodine is necessary for the production of T3 and T4, a deficiency of iodine leads to decreased production of both hormones, enlarges the thyroid tissue and causes a disease known as goitre. **Dietary selenium is also essential for T3 production.**

Of the thyroid hormones produced, about 20% is T3, whereas 80% is produced as T4 which is 40 times the amount of T3 circulating in the blood.

T3 increases the basal metabolic rate and therefore increases the body's oxygen and energy consumption.

T3 stimulates the breakdown of cholesterol and increases the number of LDL receptors, thereby increasing the rate of lipolysis.

T3 increases the heart rate and the heart force of contraction, thus increasing cardiac output which results in increased systolic blood pressure and decreased diastolic blood pressure.

It also increases the rate of protein degradation and the rate of glycogen breakdown and glucose synthesis.

T3 may also increase serotonin in the brain, in particular in the cerebral cortex.

Because T4 is converted into T3 in target tissues, the effects of T3 on target tissues are roughly four times more potent than those of T4.

Indications: hypothyroidism with T3 deficiency and overweight tendency.

T4– (Thyroxine) 6X

T4 just like T3, is produced by the thyroid gland and upon stimulation by the thyroid-stimulating hormone (TSH) released by the anterior pituitary gland.

Since T4 (thyroxine) is converted into T3 in target tissues, T4 is believed to be a pro-hormone and a reservoir for the most active and main thyroid hormone T3.

Some of the effects of T4 in the organism are: increase of cardiac output, heart and ventilation rate, increase of metabolism of proteins and carbohydrates and potentiation of brain development.

As T4 is converted into T3, this hormone should be the first choice in thyroid target therapies.

Indications: hypothyroidism with T4 deficiency, growth disorders, physical asthenia and neurasthenia, and overweight tendency. Short term treatment for depression.

Tryptophan 6X

Tryptophan is an essential amino acid which cannot be synthesized by the organism, and therefore must be part of the human diet.

Tryptophan combines with vitamin B6 and functions as a biochemical precursor for the neurotransmitter serotonin and niacin (vitamin B3).

Tryptophan is a routine constituent of many types of food such as sugar free cocoa powder, cashew nuts and walnuts, soybeans, milk and soy milk, meat such as beef, chicken and turkey; fish such as cod and salmon; cheese such as parmesan and cheddar, fruit such as bananas, and vegetables such as potatoes.

Some disorders like fructose malabsorption and lactose intolerance can cause improper absorption of tryptophan in the intestine, reduced levels of tryptophan in the blood and may contribute to cause depression.

Tryptophan has shown some effectiveness for treatment of a variety of conditions typically associated with low serotonin levels in the brain such as depression and migraines and also to induce normal sleep.

Indications: all mood disorders, depression, migraines, addictions and eating disorders.

Hormones/neuropeptides regulation chart

Hormone/ neuropeptide	Up-regulation	Down-regulation
ACTH	ACTH 6X	Somatostatin 6X TSH 6X
β-Endorphin	β-Endorphin 6X	---------------------
Beta Estradiol	Beta Estradiol 6X	Progesterone 6X
Calcitonin	Calcitonin 6X	PTH -6X
DHEA	DHEA-6X	Cortisol
Dopamine	Dopamine -6X	Melatonin4C/ Prolactin 6X
GH	IGF-1-6X	Somatostatin 6X
FSH	FSH-6X	Beta Estradiol 6X
LH	LH-6X	Progesterone 6X
GABA	GABA 6X	---------------------
Melatonin	Melatonin 4C	Prolactin6X
Oxytocin	Oxytocin 6X	---------------------
PTH	PTH 6X	Calcitonin-6X
Progesteron	Progesterone 6X	Beta Estradiol -6X
Serotonin	Serotonin 6X	---------------------
Somatostatin	Somatostatin 6X	IGF 1 - 6X
T 3	T 3-6X	Somatostatin 6X
T 4	T 4-6X	Somatostatin 6X
TSH	TSH -6X	Somatostatin 6X/ ACTH -6X

Part 2

General treatment protocols

Chapter 7

Low dose medicine general treatment protocols

This chapter will describe a few general treatment protocols for a wide variety of health conditions using low dose active cytokines, growth factors, neurotrophins and hormones.

In general low dose therapy treatments can also be combined with classic homeopathic single and/or complex remedies (*for more information consult the chapter about treatments in my book 'Cures without side effects'*) **but also with conventional medications with the aim of counteracting their side effects or in order to reduce the dosage and frequency of the conventional medication.**

The general daily dose is 15 to 20 drops in little mineral water to be taken twice a day, and kept under the tongue for deep absorption before swallowing, for periods ranging from 3 to 6 weeks or longer, or according to the particular condition and individual reaction.

The therapeutic strategy should follow the following decisional process already outlined in chapter one:

- If the pathological condition is the expression of a down-regulation (deficiency) of a certain molecule (cytokine, interleukin, hormone, neuropeptide, neurotransmitter, growth factor) the same low dose molecule will be used in order to stimulate (up-regulate) its physiological production.
- If the pathological condition is the expression of an up-regulation (excess) of a certain molecule (cytokine, interleukin, hormone, neuropeptide, neurotransmitter) the 'opposing low dose molecule' will be used in order to down - regulate its physiological production.

- According to a more 'symptoms oriented decisional processes' where the low dose molecules are prescribed to suit and to manage the particular symptoms of the disease.

Stress related conditions

Interleukin 2 –4C: general immune support during stress, 15 drops twice a day.

Melatonin 4C: neuroendocrine regulation during stress, 15 drops twice in the evening.

DHEA – (Dehydroepiandrosterone) 6X: to counteract high cortisol levels during stress, 15 drops twice a day.

BDNF – (Brain Derived Neutrophic Factor) 4C: memory and depression related to stress, 15 drops twice a day.

NT 4 (Neurotrophin 4 - 4C: modulation of anxiety related to stress, 15 drops twice a day.

Depression and anxious depression supportive therapy

Tryptophan 6X: biochemical precursor for the neurotransmitter serotonin indicated for anxiety and depression, 15 drops twice a day.

Serotonin 6X: anxiety and depression support treatment, 15 drops twice a day.

Melatonin 4C: neuroendocrine regulation, 15 drops twice in the evening.

BDNF – (Brain Derived Neutrophic Factor) 4C: memory and depression related conditions, 15 drops twice a day.

NGF- (Nerve Growth Factor) 4C: mild to severe depression, 20 drops twice a day.

NT 4 (Neurotrophin 4 -4C: modulation of anxiety, 15 drops twice a day.

GABA (gamma-Aminobutyric acid) 6X or 4C: anxiety and panic attacks, depression related insomnia, 20 drops twice a day or in the evening.

TSH– (Thyroid-stimulating hormone) –6X: thyroid stimulation in short-term treatments for depression, 10 drops twice a day.

Progesteron 6X: depression in female due to low progesterone levels, 15 drops twice a day.

Insomnia and sleeping conditions

GABA (gamma-Aminobutyric acid) 6X or 4C: to induce relaxation and sleep, 20 drops twice in the evening.

Melatonin 4C: circadian rhythm regulation, 15 drops twice in the evening.

Tryptophan 6X: depression related insomnia, 15 drops twice a day.

Serotonin 6X: depression related insomnia, 15 drops twice a day.

BDNF – (Brain Derived Neutrophic Factor) 4C: neuronal support, 15 drops twice a day.

Addictions (to be combined with the general detoxification treatment)

GABA (gamma-Aminobutyric acid) 6X or 4C: addictions to anxiolytics and benzodiazepines, 20 drops twice in the evening.

Tryptophan 6X: support for cocaine, nicotine and food addiction, 15 drops twice a day.

Serotonin 6X: support for cocaine, nicotine and food addictions, 15 drops twice a day.

Dopamine 6X: support for cocaine, nicotine and food addictions, 15 drops twice a day.

Melatonin 4C: neuroendocrine regulation during addictions, 15 drops twice a day.

BDNF – (Brain Derived Neutrophic Factor) 4C: support for alcohol addiction, 15 drops twice a day.

Huntington's disease (HD) supportive therapy

Anti-Interleukin 1 alpha (Anti IL1) – 4C: anti –inflammatory, 15 drops in water twice a day.

Serotonin 6X: mood swings and depression, 15 drops twice a day.

Melatonin 4C: insomnia and night restlessness, 15 drops twice in the evening.

Neurotrophin 4 (NT4) 4C: modulation of anxiety, 15 drops twice a day.

BDNF – (Brain Derived Neutrophic Factor) 4C: survival and differentiation of cholinergic and dopaminergic neurons, 15 drops twice a day.

NGF- (Nerve Growth Factor) 4C: neurons survival and differentiation, 20 drops twice a day.

Autism supportive therapy

Anti-Interleukin 1 alpha (Anti IL1) – 4C: anti – inflammatory, 15 drops in water twice a day.

Interleukin 10 - 4C: anti –inflammatory, 15 drops of each twice a day.

Oxytocin 6X: support for social inhibitions and fears, 15 drops twice a day.

BDNF (Brain Derived Neurotrophic Factor) - 4C: survival and differentiation of cholinergic and dopaminergic neurons, 15 drops of each twice a day.

Neurotrophin 3 (NT3) 4C: neurons survival and differentiation, 15 drops twice a day.

Melatonin 4C: neuroendocrine regulation, 15 drops twice in the evening.

Immune system support

Viral and Bacterial infections – Also preventive

Interleukin 2 – 4C: main adaptive immunity support cytokine, 15 drops twice a day.

Interleukin 7 – 4C: adaptive immunity immune support, to cause the proliferation of all cells in the lymphoid lineage such as B cells, T cells and NK cells, 15 drops twice a day.

Interleukin 12 –4C: innate immunity support, up-regulation of cytotoxic and NK cells, 15 drops twice a day.

Interferon Gamma (INF γ) 4C: immune system regulation, anti-bacterial and anti-viral action, 15 drops twice a day.

Interferon Alpha (INF α) 4C: strong anti-viral action, 15 drops twice a day.

G-CSF (Granulocyte colony stimulating factor) 4C: immune system reaction trigger, 15 drops twice a day for 3 days.

Melatonin 4C: cell-mediated immunity up-regulation, 15 drops twice a day.

Parasitic infections

Interleukin 3 –4C: immune support against parasites, 15 drops twice a day.

Interleukin 5–4C: immune support against parasites, 15 drops twice a day.

Mycoses or fungal infections

G-CSF (Granulocyte colony stimulating factor) 4C: immune system reaction trigger, 15 drops twice a day for 3 days.

Interleukin 4 – 4C: immune support against mycoses, 20 drops twice a day.

Melatonin 4C: neuroendocrine support, 15 drops twice a day.

Seasonal Flu and colds

Interleukin 2 –4C: main adaptive immunity support cytokine, 15 drops twice a day.

Interferon Gamma (INF γ) 4C: immune system regulation, anti-bacterial and anti-viral action, 15 drops twice a day.

Interferon Alpha (INF α) 4C: strong anti-viral action, 15 drops twice a day.

Anti-Interleukin 1 (Anti IL 1) – 4C: anti inflammatory, 15 drops twice a day.

Melatonin 4C: neuroendocrine support , 15 drops twice a day.

HIV supportive therapy

Interleukin 2 – 4C: immune support, differentiation and proliferation of natural killer (NK) cells and the production of lymphokine-activated killer cells (LAK cells) and active cytotoxic T cells, cell mediated immunity up-regulation, 15 drops in water twice a day.

Interleukin 7 – 4C: stimulates hematopoietic stem cells into lymphoid progenitor cells, 15 drops in water twice a day.

Interleukin 12 –4C: innate immunity support, cytotoxic and NK cells up-regulation, 15 drops twice a day.

Interferon Gamma 4C: immune system regulation, anti-bacterial and anti-viral action, 15 drops in water twice a day.

Interferon Alpha 4C: strong anti-viral action, 15 drops in water twice a day.

Melatonin 4C: neuroendocrine regulation, cell mediated immunity up-regulation, 15 drops twice a day.

Prophylaxis against vaccinations side effects

Interleukin 12 – 4C: innate immunity support, up-regulation of cytotoxic and NK cells, 15 drops twice a day.

Interferon Gamma (INF γ) 4C: immune system regulation, adaptive immunity, cell mediated immune support, 15 drops twice a day.

Melatonin 4C: cell-mediated immunity up-regulation 15 drops twice a day.

Seasonal Allergies

Interleukin 12 –4C: down-regulates IL4 driven Th2 hyperactivation and IgE antibodies production, 15 drops twice a day.

Interferon Gamma (INF γ) 4C: down-regulates IL4 driven Th2 hyperactivation and IgE antibodies production, 15 drops twice a day.

Melatonin 4C: neuroendocrine regulation, 15 drops twice a day.

Interleukin 10 –4C: chronic inflammation, 10 drops once a day.

Inflammation and pain

Anti-Interleukin 1 (Anti IL 1) – 4C: acute and chronic inflammation, 20 drops in water twice a day or 15 drops every 15 min for max 2 hours at the onset of symptoms reducing the frequency until remission.

Interleukin 10 –4C: chronic inflammation, 20 drops twice a day.

Beta endorphin 6X: pain management, 20 drops in water twice a day or 15 drops every 15 min for max 2 hours at the onset of symptoms reducing the frequency until remission.

TGF Beta – 4C: chronic inflammation, 15 drops twice a day.

Migraine and headaches

Anti-Interleukin 1 alpha (Anti IL1) – 4C: anti-inflammatory, 15 drops in water twice a day or 15 drops every 15 min for max 2 hours at the onset of symptoms reducing the frequency until remission.

Beta endorphin 6X: pain management, 15 drops every 15 min for max 2 hours at the onset of symptoms reducing the frequency until remission.

Serotonin 6X: migraines, emotional upset related headaches, 15 drops twice a day.

Progesteron 6X: PMS linked migraines in women, 15 drops twice a day.

Fibromyalgia supportive therapy

Anti-Interleukin 1 alpha (Anti IL1) – 4C: anti-inflammatory, 15 drops in water twice a day.

Interleukin 10 –4C: anti-inflammatory, 20 drops twice a day.

TGF Beta – 4C: anti-inflammatory, 15 drops twice a day.

Tryptophan 6X: sleep and depression support 15 drops twice a day.

Serotonin 6X: sleep and depression support, 15 drops twice a day

Melatonin 4C: sleep support, neuroendocrine regulation, 15 drops in the evening.

Beta endorphin 6X: chronic pain management, 20 drops in water twice a day.

IGF-1 – 4C: age dependent cartilage and bone degradation, endocrine and metabolic system support, 15 drops twice a day or mixed with neutral cream and applied to the body.

Autoimmunity

Multiple Sclerosis (MS) supportive therapy

Interleukin 4 – 4C: anti-inflammatory counteracts auto-immune cytokine triggers, 20 drops twice a day.

Anti-Interleukin 1 alpha (Anti IL1) – 4C: anti-inflammatory, 15 drops in water twice a day.

Interleukin 10 –4C: chronic inflammation, 20 drops twice a day.

NGF–(Nerve Growth Factor) 4C: counteracts neuronal degeneration, 20 drops twice a day.

TGF Beta – 4C: chronic inflammation, 15 drops twice a day.

Reumathoid Artrithis (RA) supportive therapy

Interleukin 4 – 4C: anti-inflammatory counteracts auto-immune cytokines trigger, 20 drops twice a day.

Anti-Interleukin 1 alpha (Anti IL1) – 4C: anti-inflammatory, 15 drops in water twice a day.

Interleukin 10 –4C: chronic inflammation, 20 drops twice a day.

Psoriasis supportive therapy

Interleukin 4 – 4C: anti-inflammatory counteracts auto-immune cytokines trigger, 20 drops twice a day.

Anti-Interleukin 1 alpha (Anti IL1) – 4C: anti-inflammatory, 15 drops in water twice a day.

Interleukin 10 –4C: chronic inflammation, 20 drops twice a day.

Melatonin 4C: neuroendocrine regulation, 15 drops in the evening.

Lupus erithematosus supportive therapy

Anti-Interleukin 1 alpha (Anti IL1) – 4C: anti-inflammatory, 15 drops in water twice a day.

Interleukin 10 –4C: chronic inflammation, 20 drops twice a day.

Cancer support therapy using low dose embryo preparations from Zebrafish (Brachidanio rerio)

The aim of cancer support therapy using low dose embryo homogenate preparations from Zebra fish (*brachidanio rerio*) is to induce the activation of precise gene sites with a tumor suppressing action.

Recent studies have proven that substances present in the embryo during cell differentiation are able to activate the **tumor suppressor protein 53 (p53).**

The microenvinroment of the embryo in oviparous appears to be the most effective in this kind of control. In fact this microenvinroment is quite capable of leading the stem cells to a complete differentiation.

In the course of cell differentiation, the administration of known carcinogens can't induce any tumors in the embryo, probably because the genome control system is always active.

Recent studies show that the function of the protein 53 in the embryo is to prevent malformations, to induce cell cycle arrest and apoptosis and thereby prevent tumors.

The p53 can also activate DNA repair proteins when DNA has sustained damage and it also regulates cell transcription especially during stress responses. Some authors have therefore defined p53 as 'guardian of the baby' similar to the suppressor gene.

Nevertheless, when embryonic stress is very severe and a large number of mutations are present, p53 can't repair DNA and causes the apoptosis of all cells (abortion).

These processes take place also in tumor cells when p53 is activated and this sense tumor cells are similar to embryonic mutated cells.

A recent study conducted on human colon cancer cells confirmed previous reports of an apoptotic enhancing effect displayed by embryo extracts, mainly through the pRb/E2F1 apoptotic pathway, **which thus suggests that Zebrafish embryo proteins have complex anti-cancer properties.**

To conclude, we could say that the use of embryo homogenates from oviparous fish (*brachidanio rerio*) in oncology is based on the observation that, during embryogenesis, exposure of the embryo to cancerogenous substances leads to malformations, but never to cancer, which only occurs at a later stage of gestation, when the embryo has become a foetus.

Therefore it is possible to suggest low dose embryo therapy as a sort of physiological gene therapy with the aim to regulate the proliferation of cells and normalize physiological processes and to induce the activation of precise gene sites with a tumor suppressing action.

References:

Biava P.M: Tumor cells as mutated undifferentiated cells their regulation and differentiation by embryonic extracts of zebrafish, Leadership Medica, 2001 n° 2

Biava P.M., Carluccio A.: Activation of anti-oncogene P53 produced by embryonic extracts in"in vitro" tumor cells, Journal of Tumor Marker Oncology, 1997 vol. 12 n°4

Biava P.M.: Complexity and cancer, Leadership Medica, 1999 n° 1.

Biava P.M., D. Bonsignorino, M. Hoxha, M. Impagliazzo: life-protecting factor (LPF) of anticancer low molecular weight fraction isolated from pregnant uterine mucosa durino embryo organogenesis, Leadership Medica, 2001 n° 2.

Zebrafish embryo proteins induce apoptosis in human colon cancer cells (Caco2)..Cucina A, Biava PM, D'Anselmi F, Coluccia P, Conti F, di Clemente R, Miccheli A, Frati L, Gulino A, Bizzarri M.

Guna Rerio Zebrafish (Brachidanio rerio) homogenate 4X: 30 drops in water twice or three times a day. As prevention 20 drops twice a day for 6 weeks twice a year.

Interleukin 2–4C: immune support, differentiation and proliferation of natural killer (NK) cells and the production of lymphokine-activated killer cells (LAK cells) and active cytotoxic T cells, 15 drops twice a day.

Interleukin 7 –4C: stimulation of antitumoral action of cytotoxic T lymphocytes and LAK cells, potentiate IL 2, 15 drops twice a day.

Interleukin 12 –4C: innate immunity support, cytotoxic and NK cells up-regulation, 15 drops twice a day.

Interferon Gamma (INF γ) 4C: cell mediated immune support, 15 drops twice a day.

Interferon Alpha (INF α) 4C: anti-viral action, immune support, 15 drops twice a day.

G-CSF (Granulocyte colony stimulating factor) 4C: antibody-dependent cell mediated cytotoxicity of granulocytes against tumor cells. Granulocytes (white blood cells) stimulation, 15 drops twice a day.

Melatonin 4C: neuroendocrine regulation, 20 drops in water twice a day.

Somatostatin 6X: inhibiting effect on cell proliferation, 20 drops in water twice a day.

Chemo and radio therapy supportive treatments

G-CSF (Granulocyte colony stimulating factor) 4C: antibody-dependent cell mediated cytotoxicity of granulocytes against tumor cells. Granulocytes (white blood cells) stimulation, 15 drops twice a day.

Interleukin 3 – 4C: stimulates hematopoietic stem cells into myeloid progenitor cells, 15 drops twice a day.

Interleukin 7 – 4C: stimulates hematopoietic stem cells into lymphoid progenitor cells, 15 drops twice a day.

NGF – (Nerve Growth Factor) 4C: chemotherapy induced neuropathies, 15 drops in water twice a day.

Osteoarthritis

IGF-1 – 4C: age dependent cartilage and bone degradation, 15 drops twice a day or mixed with neutral cream and applied to the site.

Interleukin 10 –4C: chronic inflammation, 20 drops once a day.

Anti-Interleukin 1 alpha (Anti IL1) – 4C: anti-inflammatory action, 15 drops in water twice a day.

TGF Beta – 4C: chronic inflammation, 15 drops twice a day.

Calcitonin 6X: attenuation of cartilage degradation and stimulation of cartilage formation, 15 drops twice a day.

Beta endorphin 6X: pain management, 20 drops in water twice a day.

Osteoporosis supportive therapy

Calcitonin 6X: inhibition of bone resorption, 20 drops twice a day.

PTH – Parathyroid hormone 6X: calcium levels regulation, 15 drops twice a day.

Interleukin 3 –4C: inhibition of bone resorption and collagen degradation, 15 drops twice a day.

Interleukin 10 –4C: chronic inflammation, 20 drops twice a day.

Skin conditions

EGF (Epidermal Growth Factor) 4C: to rejuvenate and regenerate skin, repair from sun damage, to repair wounds especially lacerations and burns, itchy and chapped skin, wound healing difficulties, contraindicated during cancer treatments, 15 drops twice a day.

FGF (Fibroblast Growth Factor) 4C: wound healing, anti age therapy, contraindicated during cancer treatments, 15 drops twice a day.

TGF Beta – 4C: persisting skin reddening, 15 drops twice a day.

Male and Female supportive therapy

Male:

Melatonin 4C: neuroendocrine regulation, impotence, sterility, frigidity, mood disorders, 15 drops in water twice a day.

Dopamine 6X: mood disorders and depression; decreased sexual arousal and lack of sexual desire, 15 drops twice a day.

Oxitocin 6X: decreased sexual satisfaction, 15 drops twice a day.

DHEA (Dehydroepiandrosterone) 6X: decreased sexual arousal and lack of sexual desire due to stress, 15 drops twice a day.

LH (Luteinizing hormone) 6X: sterility and low libido, 15 drops in twice a day.

Female:

Melatonin 4C: neuroendocrine regulation, sterility, frigidity, mood disorders, 15 drops twice a day.
Dopamine 6X: mood disorders and depression, decreased sexual arousal and lack of sexual desire, 15 drops in water twice a day.

Oxitocin 6X: decreased sexual satisfaction, 15 drops twice a day.

Beta Estradiol 6X: pre-menopause, hot flushes, preservation of pregnancy, 15 drops twice a day.

FSH (Follicle stimulating hormone) 6X: ovulatory stimulation, female cycle disorders, female low libido, 15 drops twice a day.

LH (Luteinizing hormone) 6X: sterility, low libido, menstrual cycle disorders, recurrent abortion, 15 drops twice a day.

Progesterone 6X: menstrual cycle disorders, pre-menstrual syndrome (PMS), menstrual pain and pre-menopause, 15 drops twice a day.

Gastric conditions: gastritis, duodenitis, gastro-duodenitis

EGF (Epidermal Growth Factor) 4C: gastric hyperacidity, ulcerative gastritis and epigastric fullness with pain, contraindicated during cancer treatments, 15 drops twice a day.

Metabolic syndrome conditions

Hypothyroidism

T_3 – (Triiodothyronine) 6X: T_3 deficiency and overweight tendency, 15 drops twice a day.

T_4 – (Thyroxine) 6X: T_4 deficiency, growth disorders, physical and neurasthenia, overweight tendency, 15 drops twice a day.

TSH– (Thyroid-stimulating hormone) –6X: thyroid stimulation, overweight tendency, obesity, short-term treatment for depression, neurasthenia, water retention and metabolic slowdown, 15 drops twice a day.

Hypethyroidism

Melatonin 4C: neuroendocrine regulation, 15 drops twice a day.

Somatostatin 6X: inhibitory effect on the endocrine system, 15 drops twice a day.

Weight control treatment

T4-6X: overweight tendency, 15 drops twice a day.

TS- 6X: overweight tendency, 15 drops twice a day.

Tryptophan 6X: mood and food craving disorders, 15 drops twice a day.

Serotonin 6X: mood and food craving disorders, 15 drops twice a day.

Dopamine 6X: food addiction, 15 drops twice a day.

Melatonin 4C: neuroendocrine regulation, 15 drops twice a day.

IGF-1 – 4C: metabolic system support and regulation, 15 drops twice a day.

CNTF (Ciliary Neurotrophic Factor) – 4C: appetite control, 20 drops in water twice a day.

Diabetes type 2 supportive therapy

Interleukin 4 – 4C: anti-inflammatory, counteracts auto-immune cytokine triggers, (also in diabetes type 1), 15 drops twice a day.
Anti-Interleukin 1 alpha (Anti IL1) – 4C: anti-inflammatory, (also in diabetes type 1), 15 drops in water twice a day.

Interleukin 10 – 4C: prevents insulin resistance and insulin sensitivity, 20 drops twice a day.

IGF-1 – 4C: metabolic system support and regulation, insulin resistance, obesity and high cholesterol levels, 15 drops twice a day.

Melatonin 4C: neuroendocrine regulation, (also in diabetes type 1), 15 drops twice a day.

NGF-(Nerve Growth Factor) 4C: diabetes-associated polyneuropathies, 15 drops in water twice a day.

Circulatory conditions

Anti-Interleukin 1 alpha (Anti IL1) – 4C: 15 drops in water twice a day.

Interleukin 10 –4C: 15 drops twice a day.

Hypertension support treatment

Anti-Interleukin 1 alpha (Anti IL1) – 4C: anti-inflammatory, 15 drops in water twice a day.

Interleukin 10 –4C: chronic inflammation, 15 drops twice a day.

Melatonin 4C: neuroendocrine regulation, 15 drops twice a day.

Neurological and geriatric conditions

Parkinson's disease supportive therapy

Dopamine 6X: up-regulation of dopamine secretion, 15 drops twice a day.

Anti-Interleukin 1 alpha (Anti IL1) – 4C: anti –inflammatory, 15 drops in water twice a day

BDNF - Brain derived neurotrophic factor 4C: survival and differentiation of cholinergic and dopaminergic neurons, 15 drops twice a day.

Neurotrophin 3 (NT3) 4C: neurons survival and differentiation, 15 drops twice a day.

Alzheimer's disease supportive therapy

Anti-Interleukin 1 alpha (Anti IL1) – 4C: anti –inflammatory, 15 drops in water twice a day.

BDNF – Brain derived neurotrophic factor 4C: survival and differentiation of cholinergic and dopaminergic neurons, memory support, 15 drops twice a day.

Neurotrophin 3 (NT3) 4C: neurons survival and differentiation, 15 drops twice a day.

Neurotrophin 4 (NT4) 4C: modulation of anxiety, 15 drops twice a day.

Melatonin 4C: neuroendocrine regulation, 15 drops twice a day.

Eyesight conditions

CNTF (Ciliary Neurotrophic Factor) – 4C: retinal degeneration, 20 drops in water twice a day.

General Anti-age therapy

BDNF – (Brain Derived Neutrophic Factor) 4C: memory support, 15 drops twice a day.

IGF-1 – 4C: metabolic system support and regulation, 15 drops twice a day.

Melatonin 4C: neuroendocrine regulation, 15 drops twice in the evening.

Zebrafish (Brachidanio rerio) homogenate 4X: cancer prevention, 20 drops twice a day for 6 weeks twice a year.

Interleukin 2 –4C: general immune support, 15 drops twice a day.

Interferon Gamma (INF γ) 4C: immune system regulation, general immune support, 15 drops twice a day.

Low dose medicine related websites

For any general query regarding Low Dose Therapy treatments please contact:

cureswithoutsideffects@gmail.com

Social media:

You Tube Channel:
https://www.youtube.com/channel/UC2JJq4O5F2zvFHSNPsuokvg

Facebook page:
https://www.facebook.com/cureswithoutsideeffects

Facebook Group:
https://www.facebook.com/groups/cureswithoutsideffects

Cureswithoutsideffects Blog:
https://cureswithoutsideffects.wordpress.com/

Acknowledgment

I would like to thank Dr. Jerome Malzac, Prof. Dr. Ivo Bianchi, Dr. Alessandro Perra, Dr. Jo Sorrentino, Prof. Dr. H Ibelgaufts for their knowledge and inspiration and the artist Cristina Jimenez for the artwork.

Relevant bibliography

Jerome Malzac, Materia Medica Omeopatica di Immunologia Clinica, Nuova Ipsa Editore

Ivo Bianchi, Louis Pommier, Grande dizionario enciclopedico di omeopatia e bioterapia, Nuova Ipsa Editore

Ivo Bianchi, Citochine e interferoni, Nuova Ipsa Editore

http://www.copewithcytokines.org

http://www.cytokinetherapy.org

http://www.niaid.nih.gov/topics/immunesystem/immunecells/Pages/cytokines.aspx

http://pathmicro.med.sc.edu/mobile/m.immuno-13.htm

http://www.journals.elsevier.com/cytokine

http://gunainternational.com/publications

About the Author

Max Corradi is a Naturopathy practitioner and a Life Coach. He has graduated with Honors in Homotoxicology at the Biomedic Centre in London. He also holds a Diploma in Naturopathy and Life Coaching from the Centre of Excellence UK. He has been studying and practicing the Eastern and Western traditions of wisdom knowledge, and meditation and he is also the author of Healing and Self Help books.

Other books by the author:

Healing with Micotherapy
Self-Healing with Therapeutic Mushrooms
Jaborandi Publishing

Cures without side effects
Practical healing manual of the most essential and effective
biotherapy treatments
Jaborandi Publishing

Jaborandi Publishing 2023

For more info write to: jaborandipub@gmail.com

www.ingramcontent.com/pod-product-compliance
Lightning Source LLC
Chambersburg PA
CBHW052040270326
41931CB00012B/2572